I wish to dedicate this book to my wife,
Cheryn McGillicuddy, whose love and hard work
allowed me to attain the position I have achieved
today. Also, to all the great teachers I have had
over 26 years of practice who helped me attain
the knowledge necessary to master the art
and science of sport massage.

Contents

DVD Contents   vii | Key to Muscles   viii

PART I   Preparing for Massage 1

CHAPTER **1**   Introduction to Sport Massage 3

CHAPTER **2**   Sport Massage Equipment 17

CHAPTER **3**   Getting to Know the Muscles 31

CHAPTER **4**   Preevent Massage Planning 49

CHAPTER **5**   Postevent Massage Planning 57

MASSAGE FOR SPORT PERFORMANCE

Michael McGillicuddy

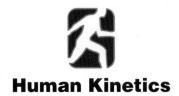

Human Kinetics

Library of Congress Cataloging-in-Publication Data

McGillicuddy, Michael, 1950-
 Massage for sport performance / Michael McGillicuddy.
   p. ; cm.
 Includes index.
 ISBN-13: 978-0-7360-8301-0 (print)
 ISBN-10: 0-7360-8301-4 (print)
 1. Sports massage. I. Title.
 [DNLM: 1. Massage--methods. 2. Athletic Injuries--prevention &
control. 3. Sports. WB 537]

 RC1226.M34 2011
 615.8'22088796--dc22

                    2010036740

 ISBN-10: 0-7360-8301-4 (print)
 ISBN-13: 978-0-7360-8301-0 (print)

Acquisitions Editor: Justin Klug; **Developmental Editor:** Heather Healy; **Assistant Editors:** Michael Bishop, Elizabeth Evans, Tyler Wolpert, and Melissa J. Zavala; **Copyeditor:** Robert Replinger; **Indexer:** Alisha Jeddeloh; **Permission Manager:** Martha Gullo; **Graphic Designer:** Joe Buck; **Graphic Artist:** Julie L. Denzer; **Cover Designer:** Keith Blomberg; **DVD Face Designer:** Susan Rothermel Allen; **Photographer (cover):** © Human Kinetics; **Photographer (interior):** Neil Bernstein; **Visual Production Assistant:** Joyce Brumfield; **Photo Production Manager:** Jason Allen; **Art Manager:** Kelly Hendren; **Associate Art Manager:** Alan L. Wilborn; **Illustrator:** © Human Kinetics; **Printer:** United Graphics

We thank the Central Florida School of Massage Therapy in Winter Park, Florida, for assistance in providing the location for the photo shoot for this book.

Human Kinetics books are available at special discounts for bulk purchase. Special editions or book excerpts can also be created to specification. For details, contact the Special Sales Manager at Human Kinetics.

Printed in the United States of America   10 9 8 7 6 5 4 3 2 1

The paper in this book is certified under a sustainable forestry program.

Human Kinetics
Web site: www.HumanKinetics.com

United States: Human Kinetics
P.O. Box 5076
Champaign, IL 61825-5076
800-747-4457
e-mail: humank@hkusa.com

Canada: Human Kinetics
475 Devonshire Road Unit 100
Windsor, ON N8Y 2L5
800-465-7301 (in Canada only)
e-mail: info@hkcanada.com

Europe: Human Kinetics
107 Bradford Road
Stanningley
Leeds LS28 6AT, United Kingdom
+44 (0) 113 255 5665
e-mail: hk@hkeurope.com

Australia: Human Kinetics
57A Price Avenue
Lower Mitcham, South Australia 5062
08 8372 0999
e-mail: info@hkaustralia.com

New Zealand: Human Kinetics
P.O. Box 80
Torrens Park, South Australia 5062
0800 222 062
e-mail: info@hknewzealand.com

E4808

PART II Applying Massage Techniques 65

CHAPTER **6** Stretching 67

CHAPTER **7** Pre- and Postevent Massage 91

CHAPTER **8** Recovery Massage 119

CHAPTER **9** Sport-Specific Treatments 149

Index   177 | About the Author   181

DVD Contents

Massage Techniques

Preevent Massage

Postevent Massage

Recovery Massage

Sport-Specific Treatments

The training DVD included with this book will enhance your knowledge of applying massage techniques. This DVD demonstrates the common techniques, a preevent massage routine, a postevent massage routine, a recovery massage routine, and treatments for some problems commonly encountered in football, basketball, soccer, baseball, golf, and tennis. The massages and sport-specific techniques that appear on the DVD are marked with this symbol in the text:

Throughout this DVD, the individual performing the massage techniques is referred to as a *trainer* for the sole purpose of consistency and simplicity. The techniques depicted can be applied by athletic trainers, physical therapists, massage therapists, or any other professionals who are operating within their proper scope of practice. It is the responsibility of professionals to objectively assess their own level of competency to perform the massage techniques and to avoid all maneuvers that would result in a violation of proper scope of practice.

Key to Muscles

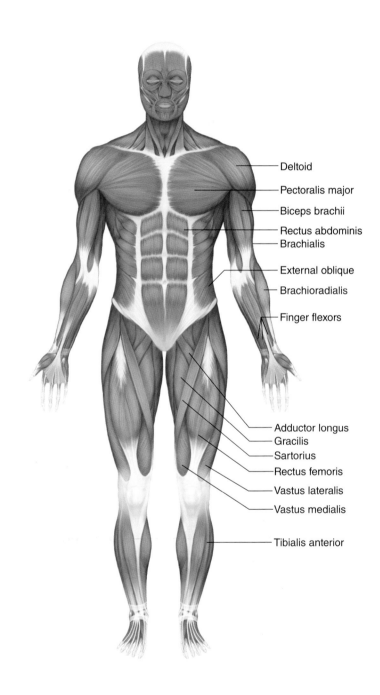

Deltoid

Pectoralis major

Biceps brachii

Rectus abdominis

Brachialis

External oblique

Brachioradialis

Finger flexors

Adductor longus

Gracilis

Sartorius

Rectus femoris

Vastus lateralis

Vastus medialis

Tibialis anterior

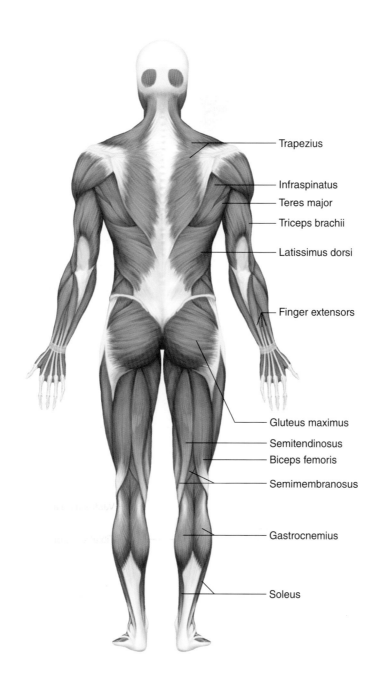

Trapezius

Infraspinatus

Teres major

Triceps brachii

Latissimus dorsi

Finger extensors

Gluteus maximus

Semitendinosus

Biceps femoris

Semimembranosus

Gastrocnemius

Soleus

PART I

Preparing for Massage

CHAPTER 1

Introduction to Sport Massage

Throughout history people have always known that some sort of touch helped human beings recover from exercise and injury. Massage has been practiced in almost every culture on earth since civilization began. It may have started with indigenous Native Americans, Africans, Australians, and Hawaiians. Records from many ancient civilizations, such as Egypt, China, Japan, and India, show that massage was incorporated into daily life. The earliest forms of Western massage were practiced by the Greeks and Romans. They built gymnasiums that incorporated massage, hot springs, and baths as part of their culture, particularly their sport and exercise practices. The Greeks first built gymnasiums to promote their military and athletic training. After their defeat by the Romans, the Greeks continued to build gymnasiums and emphasize their importance for health and social functions.

Many current massage therapy texts credit Pehr Henrik Ling (1776–1839) as the father of modern massage, and he is also considered the father of physical therapy. Ling developed his own system of medical gymnastics, exercise, and massage, which became known as Swedish massage. Ling's system of massage strokes was applied to decrease soreness, improve circulation, reduce muscle tension, and restore range of motion.

In the 1980s a man named Jack Meagher became well known as a leader in sport massage in the United States. Jack was the official massage therapist for the U.S. Olympic equestrian team and worked with many National Football League players. At that time, many in the medical professions doubted the efficacy of sport massage therapy. Jack had spent many years mastering his trade on human beings. Often, he had heard that the benefits of massage were purely psychological. So Jack decided that he would administer sport massage to horses. He wanted to prove that the benefits of massage were more than psychological. At the 1976 Olympic Games, the United States equestrian team won two gold medals and a silver medal. After the Olympic success, Jack was asked to speak about sport massage to many massage therapy professional organizations.

Through his personal experience Jack knew that professional athletes could extend their careers with the proper application of sport massage techniques. The introduction of his book *Sport Massage* (written with Pat Boughton) includes the following statement: "Whatever sport you play, sports massage will give you 20 percent extra performance, extra protection, extra time, per game, per season, per career" (p. xiii). His explanation was that the proper application of sport massage should allow an athlete to go through a full range of motion effortlessly. Often, the greatest source of limitation came from the internal resistance in opposing muscles groups as they crossed over the joints. As an athlete got older, this internal muscle resistance would increase, resulting in less efficient performance. Jack's sport massage techniques were designed to eliminate as much of the internal muscle resistance as possible. The result was that athletes were restored, rejuvenated, and inspired to continue to perform at high levels of professional sport.

Another individual of historical importance to sport massage in the United States is Aaron L. Mattes. Aaron has been an international lecturer at medical seminars and massage therapy conventions on the subject of therapeutic stretching. He has spent over 250,000 hours in sport participation, sport and health instruction, rehabilitation, athletic training, sports medicine, and prevention programs. Aaron developed a method of stretching called active isolated stretching, which he has mastered over the last 45 years. Active isolated stretching is a scientific method of stretching that isolates every muscle group of every major joint in the body. It requires the athlete to move the joints actively through a range of motion repeatedly until full range of motion is achieved.

Sport massage has evolved in the United States as a specialty modality because of many outstanding practitioners. People like Meagher and Mattes combined massage techniques, stretching protocols, and exercise to expand the effectiveness of sport massage treatments. These core principles make up much of the art and science of sport massage today.

DEFINING SPORT MASSAGE

In the United States, most states require licensure to practice massage, but state regulations vary. Some states require 1,000 hours of education, and others require 500. In all states that require licensure, students of massage must pass a written exam to obtain a license. Sport massage itself is not a licensed specialty within any state; however, a licensed massage therapist who wants to specialize in sport massage must obtain continuing education with the intent of obtaining certification in that specialty. It is usually in these continuing education programs that prospective practitioners learn about the scope of practice of sport massage.

Definitions of sport massage vary, but my definition is that sport massage is the specific application of massage techniques, hydrotherapy protocols, range of motion, flexibility procedures, and strength-training principles on athletes to achieve a specific goal. The application of sport massage requires an understanding of basic principles. By understanding those basic principles, the trainer can determine the goal of the massage and then perform the techniques to achieve it.

PROCESS FOR SPORT MASSAGE

From the intake process, through the massage, and until the conclusion of treatment, the trainer is responsible for the athlete's safety, comfort, modesty, and the effectiveness of the treatment. Most sport massage begins by having an athlete fill out some sort of massage intake information (see figure 1.1 on pages 6 to 7), such as what sport he is participating in, what part of the body is to be addressed, and what level of pain the athlete is experiencing. Informed consent is always required, so the trainer should explain what area of the body will be addressed, what the treatment is for, and what the athlete should expect to feel during the treatment.

Most forms include a full-body chart with right side, anterior, posterior, and left side views of the body to be marked. If whole-body areas are sore, broad pencil strokes are used to cover the entire areas on the chart. If smaller localized areas are painful, small dots or Xs are used on the body chart to identify them.

Before any sport massage is ever administered, the trainer should conduct a brief interview of the athlete. One of the most important reasons for conducting the interview is to determine the goal of the massage. Usually, the goal is determined by the timing of the massage. Is it a preevent, inter-competition, postevent, recovery, or maintenance massage? The trainer should also look at how the athlete has marked the intake form to determine the goal more specifically. After the goal of the massage has been established, the trainer applies all the professional skills that she possesses to achieve that outcome.

The trainer then directs the athlete to lie on the table in the best position to begin the massage treatment. The trainer should drape the athlete properly for comfort and modesty. During the massage, orthopedic assessment, strength testing, stretching, hydrotherapy, and massage techniques may be applied. Most sport massage treatments require the athlete to move the body while the massage is being administered. Oils, lotions, creams, or ointments are often used during the massage, depending on the type of

Figure 1.1   Sample Massage Intake Form

Client name: _____

Date of birth: _____/_____/_____ Check one: male _____ female _____

Street address: _____

City: _____ State: _____ Zip: _____

Phones: Home _____ Work _____ Cell _____

Emergency contact: _____ Phone: _____

Have you ever received a massage therapy treatment before? ❏ Yes ❏ No

List sports you participate in: _____

Medical Information

Check "Yes" for all current conditions that apply to you. Check "No" for others.

❏ Yes ❏ No   Pregnancy

❏ Yes ❏ No   Diabetes: Type _____

❏ Yes ❏ No   Stroke

❏ Yes ❏ No   Disc or spine problems

❏ Yes ❏ No   Bruise easily

❏ Yes ❏ No   Cardiac conditions (specify: _____)

❏ Yes ❏ No   Cancer (specify: _____)

❏ Yes ❏ No   Allergies (specify: _____)

❏ Yes ❏ No   Arthritis (specify: _____)

❏ Yes ❏ No   Hypertension

❏ Yes ❏ No   Varicose veins

❏ Yes ❏ No   Headaches

❏ Yes ❏ No   Blood clots

❏ Yes ❏ No   Osteoporosis

Are you presently under the care of a physician? ❏ Yes ❏ No

Physician's name: _____ Physician's phone: _____

What is the diagnosis? _____ Date of diagnosis: _____

Treatment Information

Please shade in areas of major discomfort. Use Xs to indicate localized areas of discomfort.

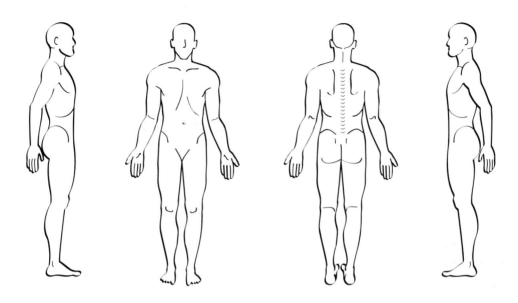

Are you experiencing discomfort (pain, numbness, tingling, or limited movement)? ❑ Yes ❑ No

If so, where is the discomfort? _____

When did the discomfort begin? _____

What level of discomfort are you experiencing? ❑ Mild ❑ Moderate ❑ Severe

Do you feel pain anywhere? ❑ Yes ❑ No   If yes, where? _____

Do you feel pain with movement? ❑ Yes ❑ No   If yes, where? _____

Do you feel pain with touch? ❑ Yes ❑ No   If yes, where? _____

Do you feel pain at rest? ❑ Yes ❑ No   If yes, where? _____

I, the undersigned, understand that a licensed trainer or a supervised student will provide the massage therapy treatment that I receive. I release the students and trainer from any and all liability because of injury or other causes resulting from the treatment. I expressly give permission for the massage session(s) I receive, and I understand that these services are not a substitute for medical care. I have stated all medical conditions of which I am aware.

Athlete's signature: _____ Date: _____

From M. McGillicuddy, 2011, *Massage for Sport Performance* (Champaign, IL: Human Kinetics).

treatment being administered. At the conclusion of the sport massage, the trainer should observe the athlete's movement in getting off the table for any signs of discomfort. Recommendations for hydrotherapy, stretching, strengthening, or any other continued treatment should be given at this time.

ROLE OF THE TRAINER

Those who provide a therapeutic service have entered into a relationship with another person where one person is in a position of power over the other. The law will hold a trainer liable for any unprofessional or unethical behavior. Therefore, trainers can provide only those massage treatments in which they have been properly trained. The trainer should protect the athlete's privacy and comfort at all times while administering the massage.

When human beings become stressed, two things usually happen automatically. They tense their bodies, and they hold their breath. This condition is often referred to as the fight or flight syndrome. If tensing the body and holding the breath is the normal reaction to stress, then the athlete should be encouraged to breathe and relax when receiving a massage. When asked to relax on a massage table, athletes usually state that they are relaxed, but when the trainer presses on a tender area, they often tense up and hold their breath. When the trainer catches an athlete tensing and holding his breath during a massage treatment, the trainer can suggest that the athlete breathe and let go in the area being treated.

Sometimes the athlete cannot help tensing because the trainer is too aggressive with the pressure of the technique. In that case the trainer needs to communicate with the athlete about the amount of pressure being used. To communicate with the athlete about the pressure being applied in any part of the body at any time, a pain scale from 1 to 10 is used. Athletes reporting a sensation of 1 would be informing the trainer of almost no sensation from the massage technique being applied. Athletes reporting a sensation of 10 would be in extreme pain. When athletes tense and hold their breath during the treatment, the effectiveness of the treatment decreases, and they are likely to report a higher number on the pain scale. Holding the breath stops oxygen from entering the body, and tensing an area restricts blood flow there. Neither situation is conducive for relieving pain or healing the body.

Staying within the 5 to 8 range on the pain scale while applying massage techniques is preferred. The higher the level of discomfort that athletes experience, the more likely they are to hold their breath and tense their bodies. Athletes who receive sport massage on a regular basis are usually in tune with their bodies. When they learn how to breathe and let go of the various parts of their bodies, they also perform better when participating in their sport because they have greater control of their bodies.

ROLE OF THE ATHLETE

In many sports, athletes may consider it a sign of weakness to admit that something hurts. In a training room, however, not admitting that something hurts is counterproductive to the effectiveness of treatment. For that reason, an honest relationship between the athlete and the trainer is essential. Athletes who will not admit that they are hurt or divulge the injury's severity are difficult to assess and treat properly. While the treatment is being administered, the athlete needs to be honest about how the treatment feels. The goal of sport massage treatments is usually to decrease discomfort in the athlete's body. The athlete needs to be honest about how much something hurts or when the pain increases or decreases so that the trainer can provide proper treatment.

A sport massage usually begins with the athlete filling out an intake form. The athlete must fill out the form honestly and accurately so that the trainer can accurately assess for the treatment. The trainer needs to know what areas are painful, when the areas to be addressed became a problem, and the intensity of pain.

During treatment, cooperation between the athlete and the trainer is essential in effective application of sport massage techniques. Frequently, the trainer will need an athlete to move in a certain way or to let go during treatment. A particular massage technique may be best applied when the athlete is in the face-up position. Another technique may require the athlete to be in the face-down or side-lying position. The athlete may be instructed to move into different positions at different times in the massage treatment. In the early stages of a muscle strain, the trainer will identify the exact site of the strain and apply a broad surface technique like compression with the palm of the hand. The athlete is then asked to move the muscle being compressed back and forth to help with the early stages of scar tissue formation in that area. During parts of a massage treatment, the athlete will be encouraged to attempt to let go or soften an area of the body so that the massage technique will feel less invasive. At other times, the athlete will be encouraged to move a muscle or joint to assist in reducing discomfort of the massage technique or aid in aligning muscle fiber.

Posttreatment suggestions for an athlete after receiving a sport massage vary depending on the purpose of the massage. If the massage treatment was for an acute stage of injury, ice treatments are often suggested, such as soaking a sprained ankle in cold water or applying an ice pack to a shoulder. Ice applications decrease the inflammatory response after the massage treatment has been administered. If the massage application was for treating trigger points or tender spots, stretching the area treated

Massage as Nonverbal Communication

From a handshake to a hug, human beings often communicate through nonverbal communication. Have you ever felt immediately uncomfortable when someone at a party or business meeting put his hands on you? Most people are sensitive to touch. We all have personal space comfort zones and touch comfort zones. We do not like people getting too close to us when they talk to us, and we all have comfort zones where we are comfortable being touched. Even if we are comfortable with being touched, we may not be comfortable with the feel of the touch that is delivered. Trainers must be conscious of the way that people interpret touch. What the trainer is thinking about, that is, the trainer's focus and intent, can enhance or detract from the effectiveness of the massage. The feeling and energy of the trainer's hands make a big difference to the athlete.

would be recommended. Stretching after treatment of trigger points or tender spots reeducates the muscles. After treatment of strains and sprains, range of motion and strengthening exercises for the area treated would be recommended. Active range of motion and strengthening exercises for strains and sprains decrease the formation of adhesions and strengthen the muscle or joint.

When athletes want to get better, they report accurately what they are feeling during treatment, they listen to the trainer, and they comply with recommendations between treatments, all of which allows them to return to playing much quicker. Athletes must want to get better when being treated. In most cases, athletes want their condition to improve because they want to get back on the field to play their sport. The will to improve helps athletes heal much faster. When they want to heal, athletes cooperate during and after treatment, which makes the treatment more effective.

KEY PRINCIPLES

Understanding what is happening in an athlete's body before, during, and after a workout allows the trainer to know why sport massage techniques are applied in a particular way. Before activity, athletes' bodies usually start at normal body temperature. Then they engage in a warm-up for their sport, which elevates their body temperature, increases their respiratory rate, increases their circulatory rate, engages their neuromuscular pathways, and gives them a psychological lift. They participate in their sport activity to different degrees of exertion and then go through a cool-down period.

The cool-down period must allow their body temperature to decrease, their respiratory rate to decrease, and their circulatory rate to slow down. The massage techniques applied at events must complement the changes occurring in the athlete's body.

Sometimes the application of sport massage has nothing to do with events; it may be more about applications for injuries. Athletes may have injuries before they exercise, or they may occur during exercise. Some injuries are acute, some injuries become chronic, and some injuries require surgery and then rehabilitation. In each of these situations, a different application of sport massage is required. Whether it is event sport massage or massage for injuries, how does the trainer determine what application would be most appropriate?

The four key principles of sport massage are timing, intent, technique, and checking results. The first key principle that the trainer must establish is the timing of the massage. The timing determines the intent, and the intent determines the techniques to be administered. After the sport massage is complete, an assessment of the effectiveness of the massage determines the result. Let's take a closer look at each of these key principles.

Timing and Intent

Timing refers to when the sport massage application is administered to the athlete. The six categories of timing for athletes are preevent, inter-competition, postevent, recovery massage, maintenance massage, and injury management. In most applications of massage, the timing of the massage is not important to the outcome, but in sport massage the timing is critical to the effectiveness of the massage. The trainer must know what the athlete is about to do, what the athlete is doing, or what the athlete has done to know what the purpose of the sport massage is. The intent of the sport massage is determined by its timing.

- **Preevent massage** is a sport massage administered right before an athlete is about to warm up for a workout or competition. The intent of preevent sport massage is to assist the athlete in warming up, increase circulation to the muscles, maintain the athlete's flexibility, and provide a psychological lift before a workout or competition.

- **Inter-competition massage** is a sport massage administered between workouts or competitions when the athlete is going to work out or compete again the same day. The intent of inter-competition sport massage is essentially the same as preevent sport massage, but because the athlete has already worked out or competed once, the trainer must consider soreness, fatigue, and any injuries that may have occurred.

- **Postevent massage** is a sport massage administered right after the athlete has finished a workout or competition, after a cool-down period. The intent of postevent sport massage is to assist the athlete in cool-down and immediate recovery from a workout or competition, relieve any cramping, reduce soreness, enhance venous return, and promote lymphatic drainage.

- **Recovery massage** is a sport massage that is administered at least a day after the athlete has completed a workout or competition. The intent of recovery sport massage is to reduce soreness, restore blood flow, increase range of motion, promote lymphatic drainage, and reestablish balance and a sense of well-being.

- **Maintenance massage** is a sport massage that is administered in the off-season or when an athlete is not training heavily. This sport massage can be deep and aggressive if necessary. The intent of maintenance sport massage is to address any chronic injuries, relieve common stress patterns, increase flexibility, increase strength, and strengthen proper neurological pathways.

- **Injury management** is a sport massage administered when an athlete has sustained an injury. Injury management includes treating acute and chronic stages of injury, pre- and postoperation conditions, and rehabilitation. The intent of injury management sport massage is to decrease swelling in tissue, reduce muscle spasms in tissue, restore proper neuromuscular patterns, restore flexibility, and increase strength and endurance.

Common Techniques

No one massage technique could possibly accomplish all the necessary intents of sport massage. Most trainers are highly trained professionals who have been educated in a variety of modalities. This section provides an overview of many of the common massage techniques used in sport massage, detailing the strokes and their effects. The most common sport massage techniques are tapotement, compressive effleurage, petrissage, friction, direct pressure, compression, broadening strokes, cross-fiber friction, circular friction, jostling and shaking, stripping strokes, range of motion, and stretching.

- **Circular friction** is applied with the thumb, fingers, or hand, using enough pressure to move the targeted tissue in a circular motion. The purpose of circular friction is to warm an area of the body, break up adhesions that may have formed between the skin and muscle, decrease sensitivity in the superficial tissue, increase localized blood flow, and increase ease of movement before activity or deeper massage.

- **Friction strokes** are applied by compressing tissues so that one layer usually glides over another. Friction strokes may be applied rapidly to stimulate or slowly to inhibit tissue. Friction may also be applied to break up superficial adhesions and warm and stimulate the skin.

- **Jostling and shaking strokes** are applied by grasping the targeted tissue and then rocking and shaking it at various speeds. Grasping is accomplished by squeezing tissue between fingers and thumbs and then performing the rocking or shaking motions. Jostling and shaking are applied as finishing strokes to stimulate the nervous system and ease tension at the end of a massage.

- **Compression strokes** are applied by rhythmical pumping motions with the hand or foot. The targeted tissues are the bellies of muscles. The compression is accomplished by trapping the muscle bellies between a hand or foot and a hard surface of the body such as bone. This rhythmical pumping action brings blood to the muscle and spreads muscle fibers. Compression strokes are often given with the palm of the hand, but they can also be given with the flats of the hands. Flats of hands strokes are accomplished by making a fist with the hand and using the backs of the fingers to make contact.

- **Range of motion techniques** are performed by actively or passively moving a joint through motion. Injured athletes are often unable to move the part of the body that they have injured. To reintroduce movement to the injured body part, the trainer applies gentle movements to the athlete's body without the athlete's engaging the muscles. Passive means that the athlete is not helping to create the movement. Passive range of motion is often used in massage to stretch and provide sensation to a joint. Active range of motion can be applied while performing other massage techniques to enhance their effects or to provide a stronger stretch. In active range of motion, the athlete assists in the creation of the movement.

- **Therapeutic stretching** is applied to the body by taking joints through a range of motion. These stretching techniques may be performed with active or passive motions. The difference in range of motion and stretching is the added force applied at the end of the range of motion. Many times the amount of range of motion possible for a joint far exceeds what an athlete can move the joint through. Stretching is applied to maximize the total amount of range of motion available to the joint. The purpose of stretching may be to warm up muscles, decrease stiffness, increase range of motion, and rehabilitate injuries.

- **Compressive effleurage strokes** are moderate-pressure gliding strokes over an extended part of the body. Compressive effleurage strokes can be applied quickly or slowly to stimulate or sedate the nerve endings. Compressive effleurage increases localized circulation by releasing histamines in the body. Histamine vasodilates the capillary walls, increasing blood flow to the area. Compressive effleurage enhances venous return and aids lymphatic movement by pushing blood using mechanical pressure. Compressive effleurage strokes should always be applied toward the heart, or moving from the distal to proximal ends of muscles.

- **Petrissage strokes,** or kneading movements, are applied by picking up, squeezing, and pressing tissue. The application of petrissage increases blood flow, milks metabolic waste products, breaks up adhesions (a fibrous tissue that forms between tissues or organs inside the body) by separating layers of tissue, affects the tonus (amount of tension) of muscle, reduces muscle soreness, and relieves general fatigue. The squeezing of muscles releases histamines, which increases blood flow to the area. Metabolic waste products are a by-product of muscle contraction, and squeezing the muscle bellies is thought to force the waste out of the muscle. Any time tissue becomes inflamed, adhesions are likely to form. Petrissage lifts muscles away from each other and the bone to help prevent adhesions from sticking tissues together.

- **Broadening strokes** are applied to the bellies of muscles with the hands together in the center of the muscles using a downward and outward motion. The purpose of a broadening stroke is to flatten out the belly of the muscle widthwise to increase its length. A muscle with more length and width contracts more efficiently.

- **Stripping strokes** are applied with a finger or the thumbs while gliding usually from insertion to origin. Stripping strokes can be applied to strengthen a muscle or to locate tender spots or trigger points in the belly of the muscle.

- **Direct pressure** is applied by pressing with the thumb, finger, palm, elbow, or foot in one place and holding constant pressure. Direct pressure increases sensory stimulation in tissue, allowing the athlete to feel a specific area of the body. If a comfortable constant pressure is maintained, the motor nerve to the muscle will respond by adapting to the increased pressure. As a result, when the direct pressure is removed, the tonus of the muscle will decrease. When the tonus of a muscle decreases, the blood flow and range of motion of the muscle increase.

- **Cross-fiber friction**, or deep transverse friction, is applied with the fingers or the thumb on a muscle, tendon, or ligament on an exact site with firm, consistent pressure and a back-and-forth motion. Cross-fiber friction is applied with enough pressure to pin the skin against the muscle underneath the application. The skin and muscle are moved in the same motion. The purpose of cross-fiber friction is to agitate the tissue mildly. This mild agitation can bring blood to the area, break up spasms in muscle, or soften the matrix of forming scar tissue so that the scar is more pliable.

- **Tapotement** (also known as percussion or tapping) is the application of quick alternating striking motions by tapping, cupping, pounding, or hacking. In sport massage, tapotement is often used in preevent massage to stimulate and bring blood to the area being treated.

Checking Results

When the sport massage is completed, the last step is to assess the effectiveness of the treatment. Many outcomes may have been intended from the beginning of the sport massage application. The intent of preevent sport massage is to stimulate and warm up the tissue of the athlete's body. (See chapters 4 and 7 for more on preevent massage.) The intent of postevent sport massage is to help relieve postexercise soreness and prevent the athlete's body from tightening while cooling down. (See chapters 5 and 7 for more on postevent massage.) Various methods can be used to measure the effectiveness of the treatment. The first is by simply asking the athlete how she feels or by asking the athlete to go through a range of motion that was difficult to perform before the treatment. The second method is to watch the athlete's movements. Does the athlete seem stimulated and ready to go after a preevent massage? Is the athlete able to get up from the massage table without stiff, painful movements after a postevent massage? Getting positive feedback is essential to establishing that the sport massage was effective from the perspective of both the athlete and the trainer.

APPLYING THE PRINCIPLES

The following scenarios provide hypothetical applications of the four key principles of massage. A trainer is providing a preevent sport massage to a basketball player. This massage is performed at the arena before the athlete's warm-up before the game. The intent of the preevent sport massage is to assist the athlete in warming up, to increase circulation to the muscles, to maintain the athlete's flexibility, and to provide a psychological lift. The order of techniques for preevent sport massage would be brisk friction, compression, tapotement, range of motion, and stretching. The trainer makes sure that he has addressed the athlete's major concerns. As the athlete is leaving the sport massage table, the trainer ends the session with encouraging communication: "You look great, and I know you are going to do well today." In leaving the massage area, the athlete looks excited and inspired. The psychological lift is as important as the techniques used in the massage.

Now consider this example: At the Boston Marathon, a runner has just performed a personal best time. She has finished the race and completed her cool-down period. She walks to the postrace massage tent for the postevent massage. The intent of the postevent sport massage is to aid recovery from competition, relieve cramping, reduce soreness and fatigue, enhance venous return, and promote lymphatic drainage. The order of techniques for postevent sport massage would be effleurage, petrissage, compression, broadening strokes, range of motion, and gentle stretching. The trainer makes sure to address the athlete's primary issues—muscle cramping, muscle spasms, and soreness. While helping the athlete off the table, the trainer asks how she is feeling. The trainer watches how the athlete is moving because she may cramp or find it hard to take the first few steps. The trainer reminds the athlete to drink plenty of fluid and not to get too hot or too cold right after the massage. The trainer then thanks the athlete for getting massaged.

As you can see, the timing determines the intent, then intent determines the technique. The proper application ensures a successful result. The rest of the book explains how to apply those four key principles. Applications for therapeutic stretching from head to toe will be described and demonstrated in chapter 6. Routines for preevent massage, postevent massage, and recovery massage will be presented in chapters 7 and 8. Finally, chapter 9, describes a few applications of sport massage for common conditions found in specific sports that will enhance the trainer's ability to provide treatment for specific areas of the athlete's body.

2

Sport Massage Equipment

Because sport massage is administered in a variety of environments, the equipment may vary considerably. Sometimes trainers work in the athletic training room or a private treatment room in a clinic or medical establishment, but they often work at an event site, in a locker room, or in a hotel room when traveling. This chapter examines the equipment and supplies needed for both situations and provides a suggested list of equipment and supplies for each. The descriptions of the equipment and supplies specify which supplies are essential in both situations as well as how the equipment and supply requirements differ for each situation.

MASSAGE TREATMENT ROOM

It is often stated that first impressions are important. When an athlete enters a massage therapy treatment room, the room must appear clean, safe, organized, and professional. Everything matters—from the size and color of the room to the look of the massage table and equipment placement. Massage treatment rooms come in all shapes and sizes. The equipment required and the decorations of the room vary depending on the number of trainers using the room and the types of massage administered.

Treatment Room Design

Treatment rooms designed for massaging one athlete at a time must accommodate the massage table and have enough space around the table to allow the trainer to maintain proper body mechanics. Most massage tables are 6 feet (183 cm) long and have a foot-long (30 cm) face cradle designed to insert into the end of the table. When massaging, the trainer must have room to move around the table. With the massage table placed in the center of the room, an additional 4 feet (122 cm) around the table is necessary. This space allows the trainer to stand far enough away from the table that he or she can lean into the massage strokes and use the best possible body mechanics. As a result, the minimum size of the treatment room should be 10 feet by 10 feet (304 cm by 304 cm). If massage is to be administered in a large treatment room with multiple tables, each table would still need an average of 10 feet of space. For the athletes' privacy, curtains or standing floor dividers usually divide the larger space into individual treatment areas.

Another consideration is the location of the massage room. Excessive noise outside a treatment room can be disconcerting to the trainer and the athlete. The trainer has to concentrate on what he is feeling and must be able to communicate with the athlete. The athlete has to relax and concentrate on how the massage feels and communicate with the trainer. Excessive noise outside the treatment room hinders concentration and communication. The location of the massage treatment room must be out of the flow of heavy pedestrian traffic. Posting signs outside a treatment room when massage is in session can be helpful in reminding people to be considerate.

Also, a light's brightness has an influence on the effectiveness of the massage. Massage treatment rooms should have a lighting system that can be adjusted. When administering a massage, the trainer needs to clearly see the areas that he is massaging. Treatment for strains and sprains requires muscle and joint testing, which is difficult to accomplish in poor lighting. On the other hand, when the trainer is applying nonspecific massage treatment such as postevent and recovery massage, the athlete needs to be quiet and relaxed. Dim lighting is preferred for this situation.

The flooring in a massage treatment room should be padded, especially around the massage table. Trainers may be standing on their feet all day, so they should wear shoes with good arch support because massage can be tiring on the feet, legs, and back. Hard floors such as tile or wood offer the advantage of being easier to keep clean and sanitary, but they are hard on the trainer's legs. Padded floor mats around the massage table help decrease the stress on the trainer's legs.

The room's temperature in a massage treatment room is important to both the trainer and the athlete. Administering massage to athletes is physically intensive work. The trainer's body temperature usually rises considerably during a massage. A treatment room that is too hot or too cold will inhibit the trainer's ability to perform properly and will be uncomfortable for the athlete. Generally, the room temperature should be adjusted to the athlete's comfort because she will be most vulnerable to temperature. If the temperature of the room cannot be easily controlled, other methods can be used. If the room is too cold, a bath towel or blanket can be used over the existing drape. Space heaters can also be placed in the treatment room. If the treatment room becomes too warm, fans can be used to move the air in the room. If space heaters or fans are used, they must operate quietly and not be directed at the athlete. Similarly, vents in the room must not blow cold or hot air directly on the athlete or trainer.

How the massage treatment room is decorated can add a look of professionalism. Anatomical charts of human muscle, bone, and nervous system are often placed on walls, as are trigger point charts and reflexology charts. In a sport environment, posters of amateur and professional athletes in competition work well.

One last consideration for comfort is having bathroom facilities nearby. Athletes should use the restroom before treatment starts, although at times the massage must be interrupted so that the athlete can use the restroom.

Equipment and Supplies

To provide the best sport massage possible, a trainer needs professional-quality equipment. The massage room should be neat and organized so that the trainer has everything he needs at the ready. A well-equipped massage room gives both the trainer and the athlete confidence about the therapy being delivered. A trainer will need the following equipment to provide massage in a treatment room. The checklist in figure 2.1 (page 20) provides an easy reference for making sure a training room is properly equipped.

Massage Table

The first piece of equipment chosen for a massage therapy treatment room is the massage table. Stationary massage tables are often used in treatment rooms and are much heavier than portable tables, but they can usually support more body weight and may come with contoured tops that allow the trainer to reach the athlete's body more easily during the massage. Generally, stationary tables are well constructed and durable, and some even have built-in cabinets under the surface for storage.

When massages are administered in a room with a stationary table, more than one trainer usually uses it, so an electric adjustable table is appropriate. Adjustable tables usually have a foot pedal on the floor that allows the trainer to move the table up and down while the athlete is on it. Table height is extremely useful in permitting the trainer to maintain proper body mechanics and in ensuring comfort for the athlete. Because trainers are of various shapes and sizes, they must adjust the massage table's height to fit their body requirements. The electric table is also useful because athletes' bodies come in all shapes and sizes as well. The trainer may need to lower the table to work on the upper body of a big athlete and then raise the

Figure 2.1 Checklist for Massage Treatment Room

- ❏ Massage table
- ❏ Adjustable headrest
- ❏ Rolling stool
- ❏ Blankets, sheets, towels, pillows, bolsters, and headrest covers
- ❏ Oils, lotions, creams, and ointments
- ❏ Biofreeze or other topical analgesics
- ❏ Medical and treatment forms
- ❏ Bolsters and pillows
- ❏ Sheets and towels
- ❏ Sound system and music
- ❏ Hydrocollator and hot packs
- ❏ Freezer and cold packs
- ❏ Weights, topes, resistance bands, and exercise balls
- ❏ Storage cabinet
- ❏ Hamper
- ❏ Disinfectants and sanitizers
- ❏ Paper towels
- ❏ Tissues
- ❏ Garbage container
- ❏ Space heater (if needed)
- ❏ Fans (if needed)

From M. McGillicuddy, 2011, *Massage for Sport Performance* (Champaign, IL: Human Kinetics).

table to work on the legs. Some electric tables break or move in the center to accommodate massage while the athlete is lying on the side or in other positions.

Stationary tables usually require an adjustable headrest. The headrest typically slides into the end of the table. They come in various shapes and sizes with different types of padding for comfort. Some headrests have clamps, while others are pushbutton. Most headrests adjust in two places: one to accommodate the tilt of the head for massaging the neck and another to adjust for the length of the neck.

Manufacturers' warranties vary. Some manufacturers give a lifetime warranty on the structure of the table and a two- or three-year warranty on the foam and covering. I highly recommend Oakworks massage tables because Oakworks tests its tables for safety and has been in the business of manufacturing massage tables for a number of years.

Rolling Stool

The next most useful piece of equipment in a massage treatment room is a rolling stool. Rolling stools are often used when administering a massage. They are particularly useful when massaging an athlete's head, neck, and feet because they allow the trainer to sit at the end of the table while massaging the head or feet instead of maintaining a standing position. Almost all massage rolling stools come with a method to adjust the height, and some have a ring under the stool that the trainer pushes in to adjust the height. For others, the trainer spins the stool to move up and down.

Bolsters and Pillows

Bolsters and pillows are important equipment to have in a massage room. Bolsters and pillows are used to support the athlete's body in different positions while she or he is receiving a massage. Simple 6- to 8-inch round (15 to 20 cm) bolsters are placed under the knees of an athlete who is lying faceup and under the feet when the athlete is lying facedown. The trainer can also buy body support cushions, which are well made and put the athlete's body in a comfortable, relaxed position. Like anything that is well made, these cushions are usually expensive.

Draping Materials

Most massages are administered with some sort of draping. Draping keeps athletes warm and protects their modesty. In treatment rooms most trainers use sheets that are made for a single-sized bed. Most sets of sheets come with a fitted sheet, a flat sheet, and a pillowcase. The fitted sheet is hooked on the corners of the massage table, and the flat sheet is laid on top. The pillow case cover can be used to cover the face rest. The athlete dresses down to the clothing that she will be massaged in and lies between the flat sheet and the fitted sheet. Sometimes a towel or blanket is then placed over the top sheet for more warmth and comfort. After bolstering the athlete properly, the trainer begins the massage. The draping is removed only from the part of the body that the trainer is massaging. Sheets can be purchased at discount department stores or from wholesale massage suppliers such as Massage Warehouse.

Weights, Ropes, and Resistance Bands

Weights, ropes, and resistance bands are common supplies utilized by a trainer. To increase the effectiveness of a massage therapy treatment, the trainer may incorporate movement, stretching, and strengthening before, during, and after a massage. Weights and bands for exercising and ropes for stretching are often used in a massage treatment. During or after a massage treatment, an athlete may inquire about how to stretch or strengthen a part of the body. By having the appropriate equipment available, the trainer can demonstrate stretching and strengthening techniques and have the athlete perform them. This method enhances the likelihood that the athlete will comply with suggested recommendations between massage treatments.

Equipment for Heat and Cold Therapy

Applications of moist heat are often indicated in massage for certain conditions. Having a hydrocollator in the treatment room allows the trainer to provide moist heat. A hydrocollator is a stainless steel container that heats water for storing hot packs. Hydrocollators have an adjustable thermostat so that the temperature of the water can be regulated. Hot packs are taken out of the hydrocollator, placed in a cloth covering, and placed on the athlete to provide soothing heat to tired, achy muscles.

In an athletic training room, trainers frequently use ice to treat an array of injuries. Athletes come to the training room from a competition or workout with sore or inflamed muscles and joints. The trainer places ice in a plastic bag and then wraps the ice bag around the part of the athlete's body that is sore or inflamed. When an athlete has an acute injury (one that recently happened), direct massage on the acute area is contraindicated. The immediate treatment for muscle aches and joint pains is RICE, which stands for rest, ice, compress, and elevate. A massage treatment room should have ice, bags, and cold packs. Ice is safer to apply to the body than cold packs because cold packs can irritate or burn the skin. Cold packs can be too cold from being stored in the freezer. Safe application of a cold pack always requires placing a cloth between the cold pack and the athlete's skin.

Oils, Lotions, Creams, and Ointments

Oils, lotions, creams and ointments are standard lubricants used in a massage treatment room. Athletes usually prefer a particular type of lubricant when being massaged. The most cost-effective way to obtain massage lubricants is to buy gallons and then pour them into smaller containers as needed. All lubricants should be stored in a cool, dark space to keep them from going rancid. Most lubricants have a shelf life of about one year.

When a trainer provides certain types of massage (myofascial massage, trigger point therapy, or working with scar tissue), he may choose to use an ointment, such as Prossage Heat, which is specially designed to allow the trainer to glide over an area of the body being treated without slipping. The viscosity, or glide, of Prossage Heat allows the trainer to apply pressure to the targeted tissue for a more effective treatment. The natural ingredients (including safflower seed oil, menthol, lanolin, and lavender oil) in Prossage Heat make the massage comfortable for the athlete and provide warmth and pain relief.

Topical analgesics are products that can be applied to the skin of an athlete for pain relief. A topical analgesic can be applied before, during, or after a massage. Topical analgesics are favored over oral medications because the risk of undesirable side effects is lower; they are less toxic to the athlete's system. Another advantage of an application of a topical analgesic is that it affects only the area of the body where it is being applied. The best-selling topical analgesic among health care professionals is Biofreeze.

Sound System and Music

Making the environment of a massage as pleasurable as possible adds to the effectiveness of the treatment. One way to accomplish this is by playing appropriate background music. After an athlete has completed a workout, her body needs to de-stress, relax, and rejuvenate. Workouts create a high degree of stimulation in the nervous system. Playing soothing and relaxing music helps the athlete psychologically enter a more therapeutic recovery zone. Massage therapy treatment rooms should have a sound system that has a variety of music available to match the type of treatment being administered. Not all massage treatments are intended to be relaxing. Preevent massage and some rehabilitative and recovery massage are intended to be stimulating. Those types of treatments can incorporate upbeat music. Music stirs emotion, and many sports require the athlete to have a high degree of emotion to perform at the highest level. Like a locker room pep talk given to inspire athletes to perform their best, the preevent massage and the background music played during the massage can help prepare athletes to compete.

First Aid Kit

Having a first aid kit available in a treatment room is highly recommended. Athletes often appear for massage with minor cuts, scrapes, and bruises. Having adhesive bandages and antibacterial creams and wipes available for such instances is appropriate. Massage is never administered to cuts and scrapes, so the trainer should cover these areas. Be sure you know who to contact in the event of a medical emergency. Personnel with specific emergency training may be available to perform emergency medical treatments or you may need to call 911 or other emergency responders.

Intake Forms

All massage treatment rooms should have medical intake and treatment forms. Before administering a massage, the trainer should have a medical history of the athlete. The trainer should have knowledge of the athlete's injuries, surgeries, and medications that the athlete is currently taking. The athlete should mark a body chart to indicate what part of the body she or he would like massaged. By looking at the body chart that the athlete has filled out, the trainer has more information about how and where to massage. The treatment forms also allow the trainer to keep treatment histories on the athlete. Treatment history information is important for training purposes and for preventing injuries. Copies of the medical history and treatment forms should be kept confidential and stored in a secure filing cabinet.

Cleaning Supplies

The equipment and space used to administer massage must be disinfected daily. Before a massage is administered and after each treatment, the table and equipment used should be wiped down with disinfectant. Cleaning and sanitizing the treatment room decreases the likelihood that colds, flues, and staph infections will be transmitted from massage. In some states massage establishments are inspected for health purposes. Cleaners, sanitizers, and laundry storage are inspected, and licenses are checked.

Supply Cabinet and Hamper

Keeping a massage treatment room neat and organized not only makes the room look better but also helps the trainer know where everything is and when supplies are running out. A cabinet should be used to store clean sheets and towels, oils, lotions, creams, cleaning materials, tissues, and paper towels. A cabinet can also be used for a sound system for music. A cabinet with doors that conceal the items stored keeps the room looking more organized.

Having a cabinet to store clean sheets and towels is important, but having a hamper in which to place the used sheets and towels is also important. For sanitary reasons, clean and used sheets and towels should not be mixed. In some massage treatment clinics, washing machines and dryers are available. In other cases the trainer bags up the laundry and outsources the cleaning.

EVENT MASSAGE

Providing sport massage at athletic events can be challenging. Each event location is different and finding suitable accommodations for providing sport massage can be difficult. The massage site needs to be close to the competition, which often means working outside. Since weather conditions can be less than ideal, proper equipment selection and preparation are essential for providing effective treatment.

Equipment and Supplies

Most of the equipment needed for event massage is the same as that needed for a treatment room, although there are a few differences. Figure 2.2 on page 26 provides a checklist of equipment for event massage. When working on the road, all equipment must be portable. The equipment needs to be organized, easy to assemble, dependable, safe, sanitary, and comfortable. The weight of the equipment and the containers that it is stored in are usually a primary concern.

Portable Massage Table

The most important piece of equipment that a traveling trainer has is the portable massage table. The number one consideration in choosing a portable massage table should be safety for the trainer and the athlete. Professional portable massage tables come in various shapes and sizes. Specific tables are designed for sport massage. Sport massage tables are usually made with sturdiness in mind. A professional sport massage table should be tested for its maximum weight capacity. A table should be able to hold at least 500 pounds (227 kg) and be stable enough not to collapse from the forces of the massage. Many sport massage techniques require the trainer to stand directly over the athlete while administering the massage. The massage table must therefore be able to withstand the weight of the athlete and the weight of the trainer pushing down on the table. Many sport massage tables are made with metal frames and legs to withstand the additional force required.

Oakworks makes a metal-leg massage table called the Wellspring that is great for use as a sport massage table. It weighs about 29 pounds (13 kg), making it light enough for travel. Table weight and size are important when the trainer travels because airlines charge extra fees for heavy or awkward luggage. The width of the table is 29 inches (74 cm), which will accommodate most athletes, and it has been weight tested up to 550 pounds (249 kg). The table can be purchased in a package that includes a headrest, bolster, and carrying case.

When massage tables are set up outdoors, the table legs are susceptible to sinking into the ground as the massages are being administered. Some table manufacturers make round plastic feet that can be installed onto the legs to keep the table from sinking into the ground. A useful item is a bag cover for the massage table. Generally, portable massage tables fold in half

Figure 2.2 Checklist for Event Massage

❏ Massage table, headrest, and carrying case
❏ Table leg protectors
❏ Table travel bag
❏ Protective coverings for table and other equipment
❏ Bolsters (optional)
❏ Tent
❏ Reception table and chairs
❏ Barrier ribbon (if needed)
❏ Signs
❏ Intake forms, sign-in sheets, pens, and clipboards
❏ Nametags
❏ Oils, lotions, creams, ointments, and topic analgesics in spill-proof and crush-proof containers
❏ First aid kit
❏ Cooler of ice
❏ Baggies and wrap for ice applications
❏ Blankets, sheets, and towels for cleaning and covering athletes
❏ Towels and hand towels
❏ Paper towels
❏ Garbage bags
❏ Hand sanitizer
❏ Disinfectant and spray bottles for cleaning tables
❏ Portable sound system and music
❏ Drinking water and nutritious snacks
❏ Proper clothing for hot or cold weather
❏ Sunscreen and insect repellant

From M. McGillicuddy, 2011, *Massage for Sport Performance* (Champaign, IL: Human Kinetics).

for storage and transport and can then be slid into a zippered bag cover to protect the table from scratches and other damage during transport. Most bags have a pocket on the side for storing bolsters and other supplies, and most come with a shoulder strap for carrying the bag.

Protective Coverings

Trainers should use packing covers, sheets, blankets, and towels to protect the massage table, bolsters, and other equipment when giving massages at an event. At triathlons, many athletes have race numbers and age groups marked with permanent markers on their legs. If the table is not covered with a plastic cover, the surface may be stained.

Tent

For outdoor events, a tent is essential in hot and cold weather to keep the athletes comfortable during their pre- and postevent massages. Tents need to be made of strong waterproof canvas because they protect athletes and trainers from exposure to direct sunlight, wind, and rain. If the sporting event is being held during cold weather, flaps for the sides of the tent may also be required. The number of trainers who need to work in the tent at an event determines the size required. A few trainers can work under a 12-foot-by-12-foot (3.7 m by 3.7 m) tent. At large events, the massage tent may be 200 feet (61 m) long.

Intake Area Materials

At an event massage, the trainer may need to set up an intake area outside the massage area to manage traffic flow and guide athletes through the intake process. The materials needed to create an intake area include a table and several chairs. Usually, chairs on one side of the table are for athletes to sit in while filling out their intake forms, and one chair on the other side of the table is for the person assigned to sign in the athletes. In some cases, plastic barrier ribbon may be needed to mark the perimeter of the treatment area to keep people from walking through it. Signs can be set up to direct athletes to the massage area.

Other essential materials in the intake area are intake forms and clipboards with pens attached. Clipboards and pens are essential because space in the massage area at an event may be limited. Athletes must be able to complete the necessary paper work readily and efficiently to keep the massage process moving along. Nametags can be useful for identifying the trainer and his or her credentials.

Crush-Proof Containers

When massage is being administered on the road, the choices for oils, lotions, creams, ointments, and the containers for storage are extremely important. The type of massage administered will determine which type of lubricant is most effective, so having a wide variety is necessary. All oil, lotions, creams, and ointments should be packed in a case that is difficult to crush and will not leak. If the containers break, the contents can leak and ruin other equipment.

First Aid Supplies

As in a treatment room, a first aid kit is essential at an event. Athletes often come to the massage area at an event with minor cuts, scrapes, and blisters. The first aid kit should have the supplies necessary to clean these wounds. Adhesive bandages of various sizes are useful. Trainers at an event should not be expected to provide emergency medical services for anything other than minor injuries. Trainers should consult the organization in charge of the event to find out what emergency services and staff are available and where they are located so that they can refer athletes with injuries to the proper place.

If the athlete has suffered some minor muscle or joint problem, the trainer needs to apply RICE during the massage treatment. At events, ice and bags must be available to treat the athletes, and all trainers working the event should know the location of the cooler and ice bags. Frequently, the event director or the medical team at the event provides a cooler full of ice. The trainer should check for these details days before the event so that she knows what equipment to bring.

Cleaning Supplies

The massage area at an event must be kept clean and sanitized. At an event, the trainer can use paper towels, hand sanitizer, disinfectant for the tables, and garbage bags to dispose of trash. Each massage table should be wiped down after each massage. At events, disinfectant wipes for cleaning the massage tables between treatments are easy to use and inexpensive. The trainer should clean her hands before touching the next athlete. Sometimes athletes come to the massage area sweaty and dirty from competing, and having hand towels to wipe off the athlete before starting the massage is advisable. The trainer should never use the same hand towel on more than one athlete. Bacteria and viruses can be spread from one person to another if the area where massages are being performed is not kept clean and disinfected. Towels should be used to drape the athlete, clean the table, and wipe off the trainer's hands between massages.

Trainer's Personal Supplies

When a trainer is working at an event that lasts all day or several days, finding time to rest and refuel can be a challenge. Providing massage is a physical endeavor that requires the trainer to expend a lot of energy. The body heats up and loses water, and the trainer may become dehydrated. Blood sugar levels will drop as the trainer is performing massage. The trainer should pack a sports bag or backpack with drinking water and nutritious snacks like fruit and protein bars. Between massage treatments, the trainer should drink a little water and eat small portions of food to keep hydrated and fueled for the work. Otherwise, the trainer can become dehydrated, leading to fatigue and discomfort. The trainer may want to consider packing a change of clothes so that she can adjust to changes in the weather. Sunscreen and insect repellant are also good choices for outdoor events.

Planning and Set Up for Event Massage

When planning for an event, each trainer needs to know who is in charge of running the massage event and what system will be used to administer massage to the athletes. Knowing the system for providing massage keeps everyone working as a team. At some events the athletes fill out intake forms and are escorted to the trainer's table. At other events the athletes walk directly to the trainer's table. If an orderly system is not communicated, the athletes and trainers can become confused and unhappy. The direction for the system may vary from event to event. Trainers may work directly for a team, for a private contractor, or directly for the event director. All trainers should have a clear understanding of what is expected, and they should agree to those terms before administering any massage.

When arriving at an event site, the first step in providing massage is setting up and organizing the treatment area. If the trainer is providing shelter, setting up the tent is first priority. After the tent is set up, establishing the location of the front desk table and chairs is next. Sign-in sheets, intake forms, clipboards, and pens must be available. If necessary, the area should be secured with plastic barrier ribbon.

After the treatment area is set up, the next priority is to install the massage table in the tent or area. Bolsters should be placed on top of the massage tables. Some trainers choose not to use bolsters at events because they must be cleaned after each massage. Bolsters and body support cushions, however, can be useful for event massage because they can assist in preventing cramping, especially in postevent massage. Next, the sound system should be positioned so that the music can be heard but is not blasting at the massage tables. Upbeat music is usually played at sporting events. The music adds excitement to the event, keeps the athletes in a good frame of mind, and helps the trainers keep up their energy and motivation during the massage.

After all the massage equipment has been set up, a brief meeting for all trainers working the event may be helpful. Everyone should be informed about how the massage event will be organized. The trainer needs to know the answers to the following questions:

- Where will the athletes be signing up and coming into the tent?
- What intake forms will be used?
- Who will escort the athletes to the massage table?
- How will the trainer let the front desk know when she is ready for the next athlete?
- How will the trainer let the front desk people know when she needs to take a break?
- How should the trainer handle any medical emergency that should occur?

CHAPTER 3

Getting to Know the Muscles

A great trainer must have great energy, great palpatory skills, and great knowledge of the anatomy of the human body. When an athlete requests a massage, whether a full-body recovery massage or a massage for a specific injury, the trainer must know what tissue to target. Should the massage techniques be directed to the skin, muscle, tendon, ligament, or joint? In this chapter we look at the various structures of the joints and what they do. We also look at the muscles to see how they function and what can cause muscular problems in the athlete's body.

ANATOMICAL TERMINOLOGY

Using proper anatomical position and directional terminology allows a trainer to accurately discuss positions of the body or locations on the body with athletes and other medical professionals. The terminology also allows trainers to record accurate information. Table 3.1 provides common terminology trainers should know. Some direction terminology references the three anatomical planes of the body. Figure 3.1 (page 32) shows the median, coronal, and transverse planes.

Table 3.1 Anatomical Position and Directional Terminology

Term	Definition
Positional terminology	
Anatomical position	Standing with feet and palms facing front
Supine	Lying on the back
Prone	Lying facedown

(continued)

Table 3.1 *(continued)*

Term	Definition
	Directional terminology
Superior	Above or toward head
Inferior	Below or toward feet
Anterior	Front side or in front of
Posterior	Back side or in back of
Medial	Closer to the median plane or toward midline
Lateral	Farther from the median plane or toward side
Proximal	Closer to root of limb, trunk, or center of body
Distal	Farther from root of limb, trunk, or center of body
Superficial	Closer to or on surface of body
Deep	Farther from surface of body
Palmar	Anterior aspect of hand in anatomical position
Dorsal (for hands or feet)	Posterior aspect of hand in anatomical position; top aspect of foot when standing in anatomical position
Plantar	Bottom aspect of foot when standing in anatomical position

Adapted, by permission, from K. Clippinger, 2007, *Dance anatomy and kinesiology* (Champaign, IL: Human Kinetics), 18.

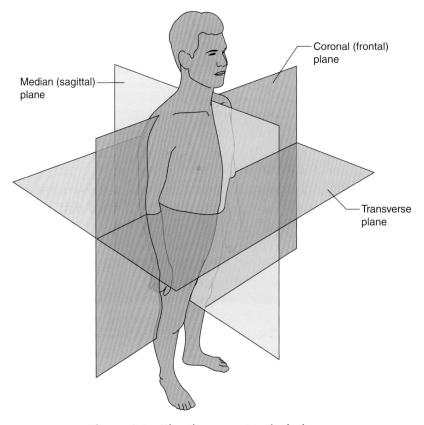

Figure 3.1 The three anatomical planes.

STRUCTURAL ANATOMY OF JOINTS

The place where two bones come together is called an articulation, commonly known as a joint. Joints allow the body to move in different directions. The basic components of joints include bones, muscles, muscle tendon units, cartilage, joint capsules, ligaments, and bursae.

Bones

Bones serve four major functions in the human body. First, they produce red and white blood cells. Second, they store and release calcium for optimum health of the body. Third, bones form the protective cage for the vital organs of the body such as the brain, spinal cord, heart, and lungs. Finally, bones provide attachment sites for ligaments and tendons to allow locomotion. Bones weaken or stay healthy because of the amount of activity they are exposed to. The internal structures of the bones change to conform to the stress they are subjected to. Without enough stress, bones weaken. With too much stress, they can crack or break. Small cracks in the bones, referred to as stress fractures, can occur from overuse.

Muscles

When muscles contract they provide movement, pump blood, and create heat in the human body. Muscles also protect joints. During surgery when an athlete is under anesthesia, the muscles lose their natural tonus, meaning that they lose almost all their ability to contract. If the arm or leg of an athlete were to be pulled during this time, the joint could become dislocated. Without normal muscles tonus, the joint ligaments and joint capsule are not strong enough to keep the joint from pulling apart.

Muscle Tendon Units

Muscles are attached by their tendons to bones at two sites, usually referred to as the origin and insertion (see figure 3.2 on page 34). The belly of the muscle is between the tendon of origin and the tendon of insertion, and when the belly of the muscle contracts it creates a force that pulls on the tendons that move the bone.

Cartilage

Where two bones articulate, soft tissue must cushion the movements between them. That tissue is called cartilage. Soft, white hyaline cartilage covers the ends of bones at most joints in the body (see figure 3.3 on page 34). Of all the joint tissue in the body, hyaline cartilage is the most vulnerable. If the pressure on the joints becomes excessive or repetitive, the cartilage can wear out. Cartilage does not regenerate, so as it wears away, bone begins to rub on bone. Bone rubbing directly on bone is called arthritis, an extremely painful condition.

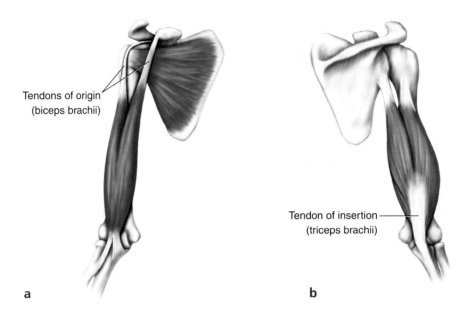

Tendons of origin
(biceps brachii)

Tendon of insertion
(triceps brachii)

a

b

Figure 3.2 Muscles are attached to bone with (*a*) tendons of origin and (*b*) tendons of insertion.

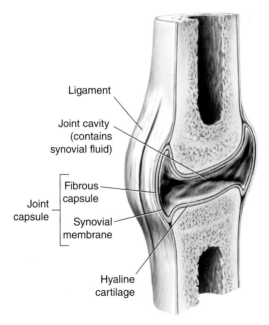

Ligament

Joint cavity
(contains
synovial fluid)

Fibrous
capsule

Joint
capsule

Synovial
membrane

Hyaline
cartilage

Figure 3.3 A joint with cartilage and synovial fluid.

Joint Capsules

Joints are held together by the joint capsule and ligaments. Joint capsules are made of tough fibrous tissue that surrounds the joint and is firmly attached to both bones of the joint (refer to figure 3.3). The joint capsules help support the function of the joint. The ends of the bones at the joint capsule are covered with hyaline cartilage for cushioning and pain-free movement. The inner lining of the joint capsule consists of a synovial membrane that secretes synovial fluid, which lubricates and nourishes the soft hyaline cartilage.

Ligaments

Ligaments (refer to figure 3.3) are noncontractile tissue that provide two major functions: They hold joints together and prevent unwanted motions from occurring at the joint. Each joint in the body is supposed to allow for a specific range of motion. Ligaments hold the bones in proper position as the joint goes through its motion, but when ligaments are damaged, the joint can become unstable. Special orthopedic tests have been designed for every joint in the body to determine whether ligament damage has occurred.

Bursae

Bursae are saclike structures that have a synovial membrane that contains synovial fluid. Bursa sacs are located strategically throughout the body to lubricate various tissues. Some bursae surround muscle tendons to protect them from excess friction, while others lie between muscles, bone, and skin. Anywhere movement can occur in the body, bursae are in place to lubricate and protect the tissue. An example of some common locations of bursae are the subdeltoid bursa (see figure 3.4), located just under the deltoid muscle in the shoulder, and the olecranon bursa at the back of the elbow. Overuse or injury can irritate bursae. If they become inflamed, a condition known as bursitis develops.

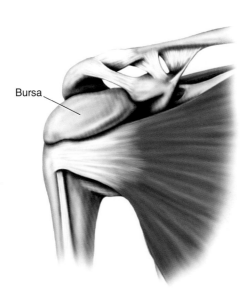

Bursa

Figure 3.4 A typical bursa.

SKELETAL MUSCLE ANATOMY

Muscles come in many shapes and sizes. Skeletal muscle is the most prominent type of muscle in the body and may make up as much as 60 percent of the body's mass. Each muscle is composed of many layers of fibers and muscle cells (see figure 3.5). The size of the muscle and the fiber arrangement determine how the muscle will function. The muscle cells consist of elongated fibers, containing threads made of myofibrils. Myofibrils contain proteins called actin and myosin. When these thin actin filaments and thick myosin filaments are stimulated, they slide past each other, causing the muscle belly to shorten. This process of filaments sliding past each other, or cross-bridging, is created by complex chemical, mechanical, and molecular activity.

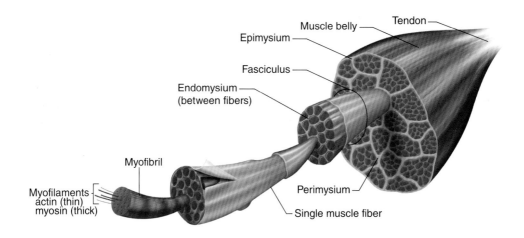

Figure 3.5 The structure of skeletal muscle.

Within the layers of a muscle are several types of fascia, or connective tissue. Fascia holds the muscle together and narrows down at the ends to form the tendons that attach the muscle to bones. Fascia also forms compartments to separate specialized tissue. The outer layer of fascia, which surrounds the outside of the whole muscle, is called epimysium. Groups of muscle fibers within the endomysium, called fascicles, are surrounded by perimysium. Within the fascicles are specialized individual muscle cells or muscle fibers, which are surrounded by endomysium. These three layers of connective tissue are continuous throughout the muscle.

Poor posture, overuse syndromes, trauma, infection, disease, dehydration, poor nutrition, psychological factors, and other influences can have a detrimental effect on the fascia. When the health of the fascia deteriorates, a binding down of the tissue can take place that potentially affects nerves, blood vessels, muscles, tendons, ligaments, bones, and organs. These painful conditions often do not show up on standard test such as X rays, MRIs, CAT scans, myelograms, and electromyography. Athletes may complain of myofascial pain in their bodies for years.

Two distinct types of muscle fibers occur in the body: slow-twitch Type I fibers and fast-twitch Type II fibers (both shown in figure 3.6). The slow-twitch Type I fibers have greater blood supply and more mitochondria (apparatus for storing fuel for muscle contraction) and utilize aerobic respiration. Thus, Type I fibers can sustain low-level muscle contractions for long periods. Fast-twitch Type II fibers provide powerful and explosive contractions, but they contain fewer mitochondria and less blood supply. Because they have less oxygen supply and use a different process for fueling the muscle contraction, they create more lactic acid and fatigue rather quickly.

Large numbers of Type I fibers are found in postural muscles and in athletes who compete in long-duration events. Athletes such as sprinters usually have more fast-twitch muscle fibers. Because genetics determines the type of muscle fibers that people have, most athletes are drawn to the type of sport that their muscle fiber type naturally accommodates. A sumo wrestler is not likely to have the same quantity of Type I and Type II muscle fibers that a marathon runner has.

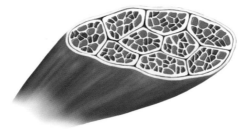

Figure 3.6 Fast-twitch (light) and slow-twitch (dark) muscle fibers.

Hypertrophy and Atrophy

One of the outstanding qualities of the human body is its ability to adapt. Muscle hypertrophy or muscle growth takes place because of reaction to added stress placed on the muscle. Placing a mechanical load on the muscle creates stress that requires the muscle to adapt. Generally, for the first four weeks (or up to eight weeks) of exercise, the muscle may gain strength, but the gain usually results from an increase in the neural-drive-stimulating muscle contraction. During this time, the person has just been learning to use the muscle more efficiently. With continued appropriate stress, however, the protein synthesis of the muscle fibers begins to change. Additional contractile proteins appear to be incorporated into existing myofibrils. This development takes place within each muscle fiber. Thus, muscle hypertrophy results from a growth of each muscle cell.

Muscle atrophy is the death, or shrinking, of muscle tissue. Muscle tissue can atrophy because of injury, disease, or lack of use. To stay healthy, muscles need constant stimulation and stress to a mild degree. When astronauts return to earth after an extended period in space, they have difficulty standing. Because of the lack resistance of gravity in space, their muscles become weak in a matter of days. The recommended treatment for back pain used to be to lie in bed for weeks. Now we know that lack of movement against gravity only compounds the problem. Estimates are that people lose three percent of their muscle strength for every day they lie in bed. If you have ever seen a person who has had a cast on a broken arm or leg for weeks and then looked at the muscle after the cast has been removed, you have seen a prime example of how disuse of a muscle cause atrophy. The calf or arm muscle that was in the cast may look half the size of the healthy leg or arm. When muscles atrophy, athletes must undergo an extensive rehabilitation process to rebuild muscle size and strength. To keep muscle tissue healthy, athletes must provide healthy, appropriate stress often.

Types of Muscle Contraction

The word *contract* means "draw together," which in the case of muscles can be misleading. When muscles contract they may stay the same length, shorten, or lengthen. The word *isometric* means "equal length." When an isometric contraction takes place, the muscle length essentially stays the same. An example of an isometric contraction would be flexing the biceps muscle to show off its bulge.

A concentric, or "toward the middle," muscle contraction is created when the tension in the belly of the muscle overcomes enough resistance to move a body segment. When a concentric muscle contraction takes place, the muscle attachments move toward each other as shown in figure 3.7a. An example would be performing a biceps curl, which you would do by having a weight in your hand with your elbow extended and contracting your biceps muscle to flex your elbow and bring the weight to your shoulder.

An eccentric, or lengthening, contraction is created when a muscle contraction allows the attachments of a muscle to move away from each other while the contraction is taking place as shown in figure 3.7b. An example of an eccentric muscle contraction would be a reverse biceps curl. You start with a weight in your hand at your shoulder and your elbow flexed. You slowly let the weight move away from your shoulder until your elbow is fully extended. The biceps muscles in your arm are lengthening as they slowly allow the elbow to straighten. When an athlete intentionally performs only the eccentric contraction portion of a weightlifting exercise, the action is known as performing negatives.

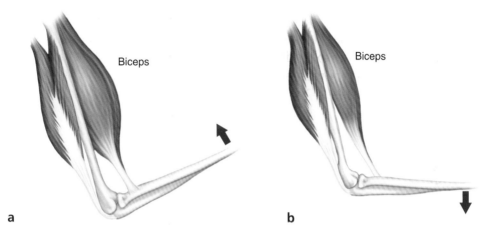

a   b

Figure 3.7 The biceps perform (*a*) a concentric contraction in a curl and (*b*) an eccentric contraction in a reverse curl.

MUSCLE PROBLEMS

A number of conditions can have a detrimental effect on muscle tissue. Learning about what causes problems in muscles helps the trainer understand how to treat the muscles.

Delayed Onset Muscle Soreness

Many times athletes are unable to work out for extended periods because of injuries or personal reasons. What happens to an athlete's muscles after she or he returns to activity after a long layoff? The term *delayed onset muscle soreness* (DOMS) is used to describe why muscles become sore after returning to activity. Good, healthy exercise stresses the muscles. When muscles that haven't been used for a while are stressed, microtrauma occurs to the tissue. In the early stages of acute trauma the body always swells. The extra pressure from the swelling of muscle tissue is thought to cause irritation to the nerves going to the muscle. The acute stage of injury lasts about 48 to 72 hours, so the muscles are usually sore for 2 to 3 days. The funny thing is that even healthy, strong people often go through this painful adaptation when they change activity and use different muscle groups. A baseball player who starts playing football may experience delayed onset muscle soreness. Fortunately, this adaptation process does not take place every time a person exercises, and it lasts only 2 to 3 days after the person returns to activity.

Strains

Strains are muscle injuries in which muscle fiber tears. Strains are graded according to severity. First-degree strains are a mild injury to a muscle that does not affect strength or range of motion of the muscle. Most first-degree strains go untreated because they go unnoticed by the athlete. Sometimes first-degree strains become second-degree strains when more stress is applied to the muscle. Second-degree strains are moderate injuries to muscles that cause pain, loss of strength, and a reduction in range of motion. Third-degree strains are the most severe and may result in the muscle completely detaching from the bone. Third-degree strains require surgery to reattach the muscles.

One of the purposes of sport massage is to prevent muscle strains. With regular effective sport massage, muscle tissue retains its extensibility, flexibility, and contractility. Extensibility is the ability of the muscle to stretch and return to normal resting length without injury. Flexibility is the ability of the muscle to lengthen up to one and one-half times its resting length without injury. Contractibility is the ability of the muscle to shorten to one-half of its resting length without injury. Healthy muscle tissue must consistently recoil, stretch, and contract as athletes work out or compete, and massage enhances all these qualities.

Spasms and Cramps

A muscle spasm is the failure of a muscle fiber to return to its normal resting length. Muscle spasms can occur in any muscle of the body at any time. In fact, most people are walking, sitting, and standing every day with many of their muscles in spasm. When enough of the fibers of a muscle go into spasm, the muscle shortens and fails to function. This condition is called a cramp. A cramp is an involuntary, spasmodic, painful contraction of skeletal muscle. Muscle spasm and cramps occur for many reasons, such as stress, overuse, dehydration, electrolyte imbalance, low mineral levels, and injuries such as herniated disks and disease.

While swimming, running, or bicycling, athletes often experience cramps, especially to the lower extremities. Cramps that occur in the legs are often referred to as charley horses. Most of these types of cramps will ease with a decrease in activity level, stretching, and massage. Another common site for muscle spasms and cramping in athletes is the erector spinae muscles that run up and down the back. The primary job of the erector spinae muscles is to hold the body in an upright position when sitting or standing. These

Pain Spasm Pain Cycle

An understanding of the pain spasm pain cycle can help the trainer decrease or eliminate an athlete's muscle pain. Pain usually starts as some form of irritation to muscle. This irritation can be caused by physical trauma, infection, immobilization, or emotional tension. When tissue becomes irritated, the athlete feels the pain and muscle tension increases. When the muscle tension increases, edema, or swelling, builds up in the tissue. This swelling decreases blood flow, which causes a buildup of metabolic waste products that inflames the tissue. The decrease in blood flow also reduces the amount of oxygen reaching the cells, a condition called ischemia. The inflammation causes a fibrous reaction in the tissue that creates limited muscle elongation, restricted joint movement, and fascial shortening. As the athlete tries to move the area of the body in pain, he or she feels even more pain and the process increases in intensity. Gentle massage and movement can break down the pain spasm pain cycle.

muscles seldom have an opportunity to rest. If they worked perfectly when a person lies down, the back muscles would relax and soften. But when you touch the back muscles of the average person who is lying down, the muscles feel tight and ropy. Sometimes they are so tight they feel like steel cables.

After intense workouts, the length and width of muscles should be reestablished by massage and stretching. Prolonged periods of heavy exercise without massage and stretching lead to less efficient muscle contraction, decreased range of motion, less power, pain, and greater likelihood of injury. Trainers should always be aware of the possibility that an athlete will cramp while lying on a massage table. Most cramps can be relieved with the application of therapeutic stretching, but when an athlete experiences cramping in more than one muscle group, medical attention may be required. Cramping in more than one muscle group can be the sign of severe dehydration and should be addressed by the proper medical personnel.

Injuries and Scar Tissue

When muscle cells are damaged because of injury, they are dead and gone forever. Muscle cells are genetically too complicated for replacement cells to grow, so the body developed the ability to create scar tissue. Scar tissue begins to form when cells are damaged, and the contents of the cell walls leak out into the interstitial space. Whole proteins from inside the cells walls attract water to the area, resulting in swelling. Usually enough swelling occurs in the first five minutes of an injury to provide the necessary foundation for scar tissue formation, but the body continues to swell in the injured area. The excess swelling can cause secondary cell damage, called hypoxic injury, which can cause more damage than the original injury. Hypoxic injury occurs because oxygen cannot reach the healthy cells around the injured site.

The application of ice to the injured area is extremely important during the acute stage of injury to help put the healthy cells into a lower metabolic state that reduces the need for oxygen. Ice needs to remain applied to the injured area for at least 30 minutes to lower the metabolism of healthy cells. When the metabolism of healthy cells is reduced, they need less oxygen to survive.

Soon after the injury occurs, white blood cells called macrophages surround the tissue of the dead cells and begin to dissolve it. This process can be felt around an injured area because it often becomes warmer than the surrounding healthy tissue. After the macrophages do their job, fibroblasts string together protein strands and inject them into the fluid in the injured area. These protein strands wind around each other and become the basis of scar tissue formation. As the protein strands form, the injured muscles should be taken through their proper range of motion so that the strands align with the direction of the muscle fibers. When scar tissue begins to form, it can stick all tissue in the immediate area together, causing a scar that can inhibit proper movement. The scar may cause additional irritation or reoccurring injury.

Applying mild cross-fiber friction at the site of the injury softens the scar tissue as it is forming, helping it become more pliable. Moving the injured muscle helps align the scar tissue in the direction in which the muscle fibers move. Icing after applying cross-fiber friction helps prevent excessive inflammation of the injured area.

One of the last stages of scar tissue formation occurs when the body injects ground substance into the scar tissue to give it greater strength. From the onset of a muscle strain, six to eight weeks may be required before the scar tissue is healthy enough to undergo extensive muscular contraction without reinjury.

JOINT MOVEMENT

Skeletal muscles cross over the joints to provide locomotion, or movement. When the muscles on one side of the joint contract and shorten, the muscles on the opposite side must inhibit and lengthen for the joint to move (refer to figure 3.7 on page 39). The joint moves in the direction of the contracted muscles. A smooth, controlled motion requires a coordinated contraction between the concentric and eccentric muscles crossing the joint. To move the joint in the opposite direction, the muscles that were inhibited now contract and the contracted muscles are inhibited. Muscle contractions may be used to speed up body movements to create acceleration, or they may be used to slow down body movements to create deceleration. Both acceleration and deceleration place extra stress on the muscles. It is during acceleration or deceleration that athletes often strain or injure their muscles.

The force of a muscle pulling on a joint is created by the contraction of the muscle. The amount of force generated by the contraction depends on the number of fibers recruited. For example, if you hold a bowling ball in one hand and a ballpoint pen in the other, you would feel the difference in the number of fibers required to contract the muscles in each arm.

The field of kinesiology (the study of motion in the human body) uses the following four terms to explain various muscle functions at a joint: agonist, antagonist, synergist, and stabilizer. When any joint in the body goes through a range of motion, the muscle that is primarily responsible for that motion is called the agonist. For every agonist muscle there is always a muscle that works in direct opposition, called an antagonist. Muscles that assist a range of motion are called synergists, and muscles that hold joints steady are called stabilizers. For any given sport activity, such as running, jumping or throwing, muscles crossing over the joints of the body must perform one of the four functions and the muscles change functions as the body goes through the range of motion.

Most athletes are unaware of the internal resistance that builds within the opposing muscle groups as joints go through motions and begin to fatigue. The more the muscle fatigues, the greater the spasming is. The more the muscle spasms, the greater the resistance is across the joints in the athlete's body. One of the reasons for applying sport massage is to reduce the tension within the muscle groups that cross over joints in the body. An athlete should be able to go through a full range of motion effortlessly. When athletes have freedom of motion without pain, they enjoy working out and competing more.

Muscle Pairings

Trainers should know which of the paired muscles crossing over each joint is stronger than its counterpart. When muscles are stronger on one side of the joint than the other, the range of motion of the joint will always tend to shorten in the direction of the stronger muscle group. If a sport requires repetitive motions of a joint, then the weaker muscles across the joint will fatigue quicker. As muscles fatigue, they have a tendency to go into spasm and eventually cramp. The stronger muscles across the joint can then pull on the spasming muscles, causing muscle strains. On page 44, table 3.2 provides a list of stronger and weaker muscles for muscles on opposite sides of various joints.

Table 3.2   Stronger and Weaker Muscles at Joints

Stronger muscles	Weaker muscles
Calf muscles (gastrocnemius and soleus)	Shin muscles (tibialis anterior)
Anterior thigh muscles (quads)	Posterior thigh muscles (hamstrings)
Hip extensors (gluteus maximus)	Hip flexors (psoas and iliacus)
Back muscles (erector spinae)	Abdominal muscles (rectus abdominis and obliques)
Chest muscles (pectoralis major)	Midback (middle trapezius and rhomboids)
Internal rotators of the shoulder (latissimus dorsi, teres major, pectoralis major, subscapularis, and anterior deltoid)	Lateral rotators muscles of the shoulder (infraspinatus, teres minor, and posterior deltoid)
Elbow flexors (biceps and brachialis)	Elbow extensors (triceps)
Forearm flexors	Forearm extensors
Forearm supinators	Forearm pronators
Wrist flexors	Wrist extensors

Knowing the strong verses weak muscles across joints allows a trainer to suggest the proper stretching and strengthening protocols for athletes. In most cases the trainer would want to stretch strong, shortened muscles and strengthen weak muscles. With the shoulder, however, the trainer always wants to strengthen and stretch the lateral rotators to prevent injury. The lateral rotators are always weaker and tighter than the medial rotators.

Another important point about understanding strong muscles verses weak muscles across joints is how the relationship affects posture and the health of the muscle tissue itself. In the upper body the pectoralis major muscle in front is always stronger than the middle trapezius and rhomboids in back. This shortening of the muscles on the front side of the body stretches the muscles on the posterior side, which is the primary reason for the rounded shoulder position of the upper body. Muscles do not function well when they are held in either the shortened position or the stretched position for long periods. Congestion from the shortened pectoralis muscle and the tightened middle trapezius and rhomboids from persistent stretching decreases blood flow to the muscles.

Chronic decrease in blood flow can cause a buildup of metabolic waste products in muscles, which is a primary cause of trigger point formation in muscle tissue. Trigger points are localized areas of tenderness in muscle tissue that cause pain when pressured, but the pain may be felt in a location adjacent to the actual source. This occurrence is known as referred pain, and each muscle has a pain referral pattern. Some patterns are localized to the trigger point in the muscle, and some are distal to the trigger points. Each muscle in the body can form multiple trigger points with various referred pain patterns. The constant recurring stress placed on muscles by being in either the shortened position or the stretched position can cause them to become diseased over a long period. Trainers need to know the importance of muscle balance in the body. Maintaining a healthy muscular balance from front to back, side to side, and to the rotational muscles of the body is critical for the health of the muscles.

Enthesopathy is a disease process at musculotendinous junctions or where tendons and ligaments attach into bones or joint capsules. Enthesopathy is characterized by local tenderness and may, in time, develop into enthesitis. Enthesitis is a traumatic disease that occurs at the insertion of muscles where recurring muscle stress provokes inflammation that leads to fibrosis and calcification.

Ranges of Motion

Every joint in the body has a certain number of ranges of motion that it is supposed to go through. On page 46, table 3.3 provides an explanation of the common ranges of motion or movements that occur at joints. The number of ranges of motion for every joint will always be an even number because a joint must always work in two directions. The following are the major joints of the body and the number and type of ranges of motion they go through:

- Toe—four ranges of motion: flexion, extension, abduction, and adduction.
- Ankle—four ranges of motion: dorsiflexion, plantarflexion, inversion, and eversion.
- Knee—four ranges of motion: flexion, extension, internal or medial rotation, and external or lateral rotation.
- Hip—six ranges of motion: flexion, extension, abduction, adduction, internal or medial rotation, and external or lateral rotation.
- Spine—six ranges of motion: flexion, extension, rotation right, rotation left, lateral flexion or side bending right, and lateral flexion or side bending left.

- Scapula—six ranges of motion: elevation, depression, protraction, retraction, upward rotation, and downward rotation.
- Shoulder joint—six ranges of motion: flexion, extension, abduction, adduction, internal or medial rotation, and lateral or external rotation.
- Elbow—two ranges of motion: flexion and extension.
- Forearm—two ranges of motion: supination and pronation.
- Wrist—four ranges of motion: flexion, extension, abduction or radial flexion, and adduction or ulnar flexion.
- Finger—four ranges of motion: flexion, extension, abduction, and adduction. (The hands can achieve a movement that the feet cannot. In the hand, the thumb and little finger can curl to meet and touch each other, a range of motion called opposition.)

Table 3.3 Joint Movements

Action	Movement	Example
Flexion	Bending, folding of a joint	Elbow is bent at start of push-up.
Extension	Straightening of a joint	Elbow straightens when in a push-up position.
Abduction	Moving away from center	Arms and legs move away from body in a jumping jack.
Adduction	Moving toward center	Arms and legs move toward body in a jumping jack.
External rotation	Rotating outward	Shoulder joint rotates externally to throw a baseball.
Internal rotation	Rotating inward	Shoulder joint rotates internally to place the hand on the hip.
Inversion	Bottom of feet turning inward	Ankle rolls inward.
Eversion	Bottom of feet turning outward	Ankle rolls outward.
Supination	Forearm turning so that palm of hand is face up	Forearm (usually) turns faceup when using a screwdriver to tighten a screw.
Pronation	Forearm turning so that palm is face down	Forearm (usually) turns facedown when using a screwdriver to loosen a screw.
Plantarflexion	Pointing the foot	Feet pointing toward the ground when performing calf raises.
Dorsiflexion	Flexing the foot	Rocking back on heels, lifting forefoot.

Adapted, by permission, from J.G. Haas, 2010, *Dance anatomy* (Champaign, IL: Human Kinetics), 3.

Knowing all the ranges of motion of the major joints of the body is one of the first steps in being able to assess the proper functioning of an athlete's body. A trainer needs to know every direction a joint can move and how it should go through a range of motion. A big part of assisting an athlete in enhancing performance and preventing injuries is maximizing range of motion, although excessive range of motion in a joint can also be a serious problem. Joints with too much flexibility can become unstable and prone to sprains. If ligaments become stretched, the muscles crossing over the joint must be strengthened to help prevent sprains to the joint.

QUALITY TOUCH AND TISSUE TEXTURE

A survey conducted among trainers asked this question: How long does it take a trainer getting a massage from another trainer to know whether the massage is going to be a good one? The answer: within a few seconds. That result may seem amazing to those not familiar with massage, but an experienced trainer can almost instantaneously recognize a quality touch.

Quality touch comes with years of experience. A trainer must know the anatomy of the body to give a good massage, but quality of touch comes from how much care and skill the trainer applies. When athletes receive massage from various trainers, they cannot help but compare the quality of touch from one to another. Quality of touch is not dependent on years or practice or high education levels. Sometimes, quality of touch is like a god-given gift that certain people possess. Trainers can develop quality touch with education and practice, but some people have it from the very beginning.

Part of quality touch comes from the energy of the trainer. The other part comes from the trainer's ability to sense what she or he is feeling in the athlete's body and then to apply the appropriate massage technique. Muscles, whether healthy or dysfunctional, have a certain feel or texture to them. Being able to sense or feel the texture of tissue is critical to providing an effective massage.

What should healthy muscle tissue feel like? The answer is simple: Healthy muscle tissue should feel smooth and consistent. The important qualities of healthy muscles are extensibility, flexibility, and contractibility. Muscles that possess those qualities feel more elastic–unhealthy muscles feel more plastic. A good trainer can sense the plastic feeling in the muscle tissue and tries work with the tissue to restore the healthier elastic consistency.

Here are some other textures in tissue that a trainer should be able to sense. When an injury takes place in a muscle, swelling of the tissue always follows. The excess fluid in the tissue usually makes the muscle feel mushy or spongy. When only a few strands of a muscle are injured, the muscle feels stringy, like plucked guitar strings. When the entire muscle is sore or overused, the whole muscle feels thick and inflexible. When muscles detach from the bone, they can ball up, creating a Popeye effect.

Besides knowing texture, the trainer needs to know how the muscles are layered. An example would be the midback area of the body. The first tissue the trainer touches is the skin. It could feel hot, cold, oily, dry, stiff, or thick. The next layer of tissue would be the middle trapezius muscle, whose fibers align horizontally to the spine. The layer of muscle tissue under the trapezius is the rhomboids. Those fibers align at a 45-degree angle to the spine. The layer of muscle under the rhomboids is the erector spinae, and those muscle fibers align vertically to the spine. While performing the massage, the trainer senses muscle texture and fiber alignment of tissue to determine the appropriate massage technique for each muscle.

CHAPTER 4

Preevent Massage Planning

The primary purpose of preevent massage is to assist an athlete in preparing for a competition or workout at an event site. A preevent massage is never meant to replace an athlete's warm-up. The pace of the massage is always upbeat and rhythmical, and it lasts no longer than 15 minutes. The massage targets the muscles that the athlete will use in his or her sport. The emphasis should be placed on warming up the superficial tissue, increasing blood flow to the muscles used in the sport, moving joints through their proper range of motion, easing any excess tension in the athlete's body, and providing a psychological lift before the completion. In a scene from the movie *Rocky*, Rocky climbed the 72 stone steps in front of the entrance of the Philadelphia Museum of Art during one of his workouts while the theme song played loudly in the background. Some viewers get goose bumps just watching that scene. That emotion is an example of the psychological lift that a preevent massage is meant to provide to the athlete.

Care should be given not to bring too much attention to sore or painful areas on the athlete's body and to avoid applying techniques that could irritate or inflame tissue. Slow, long gliding strokes should never be incorporated in preevent massage because they tend to sedate the athlete. The purpose of preevent massage is to stimulate the athlete's body and leave the athlete inspired to perform his best.

CONTRACTING FOR EVENT MASSAGE

The first step in providing preevent sport massage is securing the right to work at the event from the sponsoring organization. A trainer cannot just show up at an event, set up a massage table, and start massaging athletes. Usually, a written contract is agreed to between the sponsoring organization and the entity providing the massage at the event. This written agreement fulfills the legal obligation of having an establishment license to perform massage at the event. Professional and college teams often have trainers who travel with the team year round. Most states have exemptions for trainers who travel with sport teams. Some individual athletes or teams have sponsoring organizations that hire trainers to work on the athletes or team members. The team sets up a tent at an event, and the trainer works in the tent only on those people who are on the sponsor's team.

Providing massage in a professional manner at an event requires a lot of planning. The contract should contain all the major considerations for providing massage at the event, including the following:

- **For how many days is the event being conducted?** The duration of the event is important to know because the longer the event runs, the greater is the number of trainers needed to provide massage. Making the preevent massages available to the athletes when they need them is crucial to the success of the massage. Most athletes will not want to stand around for a long time to receive a 15-minute preevent massage, so knowing how many trainers are needed is essential to providing massage in a timely manner.

- **How many athletes are competing, and how many hours will massage be offered?** The number of trainers needed to provide adequate service depends on how many hours a day massage will be available and how many athletes will be competing. Additionally, if a sporting event is scheduled for the entire day, trainers must arrive early and set up to provide preevent massage. If the event requires the athletes to compete multiple times during the day, trainers need to be available for massage between competitions and for postevent massage (see chapter 5 for more on postevent massage).

- **Where will the massages be administered?** If massages will be given outside, the weather for the event days will be important. Events can occur on cold, rainy days or extremely hot, dry days. The athletes should be under a protective roof. Without a roof overhead the athletes might have to lie in direct sunlight or could get soaking wet should it start to rain. Neither case is conducive to massage. A tent or an open-air structure with a roof is adequate. At most large events the promoter provides these structures. In cold weather, athletes should be provided a blanket. In hot conditions fans to move the air are helpful.

- **What happens if a medical emergency arises during a sport massage?** Massage is defined as manipulation of the soft tissue of the human body. Nowhere does that definition state that the purpose of a trainer is to provide emergency medical treatment. A trainer working at an event should know what role she is to play in providing services to the athletes. Athletes can suffer from severe dehydration, hyperthermia, hypothermia, shock, heart attacks, and other conditions. Any time a medical emergency exists at an event, the professionals trained to handle emergency medical services should be the ones that handle the situation. Trainers should know beforehand what other medical services are available and where they will be situated in case an athlete needs them. The trainer needs to know whether doctors, nurses, or emergency medical techs are on hand and how to get their attention and assistance when necessary.

- **How are the trainers being paid?** How the trainers are being paid is important. The sponsoring organization may pay for the trainers, the competitors may pay, a corporate sponsor may pay, or the trainers may be paid because they are a part of a team's organization.

LOGISTICAL AND RECORD-KEEPING PREPARATIONS

Every event is different, so having an orderly system for providing massage is critical to keeping everyone happy. Trainers and athletes can become upset if things are not done in an organized and professional manner. At some events, appointment times may be required. Other events use a sign-in sheet, and massage is done on a first-come basis. Keeping unwanted people away from where the massages are being administered is also important. Athletes like their privacy, and trainers need to keep unnecessary people out of the way to do a good job.

To provide a safe, effective preevent sport massage, the person providing the massage ideally should have done an on-site inspection of the place where the massages are being administered before the event takes place. Some of the considerations for the site of preevent sport massage are whether the massages will be administered indoors or outdoors, how the athletes will know how to find the massage area and what time they should arrive, what kind of attire they should wear, and how long they should allow for the massage before competition.

Keeping accurate records of preevent massages allows the trainer to know the athlete's preferences. When the trainer provides preevent massages at many different events, keeping records allows him to learn quickly which treatments are required for each sport. Maintaining records also allows a trainer to compile statistics on the number of athletes treated and common areas treated for each sport.

The trainer should have an intake form (such as the one in chapter 1) with a full-body chart for the athlete to mark before the massage is administered. The intake form should be brief. Athletes do not like to spend long periods filling out paperwork to receive their massages. The forms should be simple, and the charts should be easy to fill out. A space for the name of the athlete, the sport in which the athlete is participating, and the area of the body to be addressed is appropriate.

A common full-body chart will have a front, back, and both sides of the body for the athlete to mark. Having an outline of the full body makes it easy for the athlete to mark what area he or she wants preevent massage concentrated on. If the athlete marks little Xs or Os specifically on an area, the trainer should inquire whether the athlete has an injury. Although the trainer should be aware of any injuries to prevent discomfort during the massage, he should provide only minimal attention to an injury. Preevent massage is intended to assist an athlete in warming up, not to treat injuries. Too much attention to the injuries may cause the athlete to be distracted by minor aches and pains prior to a competition. Bringing the athlete's attention to sore areas or injuries right before a workout or competition is counterproductive to the intention of preevent massage.

APPROPRIATE MASSAGE TIMING

Let's assume that the trainer has prepared for the event properly and is now ready to provide preevent massage. The first consideration is when to perform preevent massage. The timing depends on what kind of sport the athlete is competing in. Some sports require the athlete to make an immediate quick response, such as a sprinter who must explode from the blocks at the sound of a gun going off. Other sports like boxing require the athlete to be as loose as possible to avoid suffering a knockout early in the first round of a fight. A boxer is often still getting his neck and shoulders massaged as he takes instruction from the referee before the fight starts. But a trainer would not want to be doing that to a runner just before the start of a race because the runner's reaction time would likely be slower. Preevent massage prepares the athlete for the competition. Knowing the reaction time needed in the sport is essential to providing an effective massage.

Another consideration is whether a preevent massage should be administered before or after the athlete warms up. To determine this, the trainer needs to understand the physiological effects of a proper warm-up. An athlete often bounces around a little bit, does a few simple stretches, and then claims to be warmed up. A proper warm-up increases the athlete's heart rate, increases the respiratory rate, elevates body temperature, and prepares the neurological pathways for activity. The best warm-ups are direct warm-ups that involve doing the activity required for the sport in a minimum capacity. An athlete is usually not warmed up unless she is perspiring. Doing a proper warm-up usually takes about 10 to 15 minutes.

If the effects of a good warm-up are an increase in heart rate, an increase in respiratory rate, and an increase in body temperature, what would happen to those effects if an athlete lies down for 10 to 15 minutes while receiving a preevent massage? The effects of the warm-up would be lost. In most cases a preevent massage should be done before the athlete warms up.

PREEVENT MASSAGE INTERVIEW

Before beginning the preevent massage, the trainer should conduct a brief interview. Asking a few questions before the massage starts allows the trainer to hear the athlete's voice and tonality. Some athletes become extremely nervous right before a competition, and the trainer can pick up the nervousness by listening to how the athlete responds to the preevent interview questions. If the trainer recognizes that the athlete is nervous, the trainer should assure the athlete that the preevent massage will help in preparing for the competition. Athletes are normally a bit nervous before a competition, and the feeling of the preevent massage can divert their attention from the nervousness. Some common questions to use in the interview include the following:

- **Have you ever had a preevent massage?** The trainer asks this question to find out whether the athlete knows what to expect from the massage, whether he has a preference about how the preevent massage is done, what massage techniques she or he is used to receiving, and where the athlete wants the preevent massage directed on the body. Many athletes are superstitious. They may have a favorite shirt or socks that they wear for luck, and their preevent routines may be very specific. Anything that the trainer does to change the athlete's routine could be interpreted by the athlete as a negative experience or an excuse for poor performance.

- **How long before your competition?** A preevent massage should always be performed with enough time to allow the athlete to warm up properly before competing. Preevent massage does not take the place of a proper warm-up.

- **What areas of your body would you like me to concentrate on?** Some athletes want only minor things done to them before an event. They may be concerned with only one part or area of the body. Just a few minutes of rubbing a shoulder or ankle or stretching the athlete can make the person very happy. The trainer should be sure not to overdo a preevent massage. She may be the last person to help an athlete just before the competition, so the trainer may be asked to do simple little things to help the athlete feel comfortable.

- **Do you know of any areas of your body where you usually feel tension before you compete?** Athletes are usually in tune with their bodies and know exactly what bothers them before a competition. The trainer can easily receive directions from the athlete about exactly where to work.

The trainer should start the massage by telling the athlete, "If anything I do causes you to become uncomfortable, please tell me." Then he can say, "I can always stop or change what I am doing to because my number one goal is to have you leave the massage table feeling as good as possible for your event." Many athletes do not know that they have a say in how they are being treated. If the trainer does not assure the athlete that his input is essential in the treatment, the athlete often says nothing. Without the athlete's input, the effectiveness of the preevent massage is often diminished.

The trainer should finish the massage with range of motion or gentle stretches to help the athlete prepare for the warm-up. Preevent massage techniques assist in warming up tissue, increasing blood flow, and reducing discomfort before exercise. Range of motion and stretching prepare the joints and muscles for movement. Range of motion helps decrease tension in the joints and helps lubricate them. Stretching helps elongate the muscle tissue, increase blood flow to the muscle, and decrease excess tension within the muscle.

FOCUS OF THE PREEVENT MASSAGE

A preevent massage is usually not more than 10 or 15 minutes in duration and frequently is administered through clothing. While providing the massage, the trainer should be talking to the athlete in an encouraging way. Telling athletes that they look great, that their muscles feel good, and that they seem well prepared for competition can be as encouraging as the massage. If athletes seem nervous, the trainer can encourage them to talk to help dissipate the nervousness but should try to discourage them from talking negatively about themselves or the competition. Understanding the athletes is important. Athletes prepare for their events in different ways. Some like to sit quietly to prepare for competition; others have a lot of nervous energy and are talkative and active right before competing. The trainer should observe what each athlete's needs are and not interfere in the process of getting ready.

The trainer wants the athlete to leave the massage table feeling good and prepared to compete, not lethargic or about to fall asleep. The pace of the massage should be stimulating and brisk. The trainer wants to bring warmth to the superficial tissue of the body and increase blood flow to the deeper muscles. A good approach is to run the joints through their ranges of motion to increase lubrication and then to stretch the muscles gently.

The general rule of preevent massage is that the closer the massage is to the time of competition, the less invasive it should be. The trainer never wants to take the chance of injuring or pulling a muscle on an athlete right before the competition. Applying deep tissue massage or vigorously stretching an athlete right before the competition is often too much of a change for the body to handle. In most preevent massages no oil or lubricant is applied to the body because it can clog the pores in the skin, making it difficult for the athlete to sweat. In sports such as wrestling, an oily body would give the athlete an unfair advantage.

The trainer should have a preevent routine for the upper body and the lower body. Preevent massage is not intended to be applied to the entire body. The trainer wants to target the muscles used in the athlete's sport. An upper-body preevent massage should include these techniques:

- Friction to create heat to warm up the superficial tissue of the back
- Compression to increase blood flow to the muscles of the back and arms
- Shaking or rocking of the arms and shoulders to decrease excess tension
- Tapotement to stimulate the muscles of the arm and shoulder
- Range of motion of the arm and shoulder joints to increase or decrease stiffness
- Gentle stretching to prepare muscles for the warm-up

A lower-body preevent massage should include these techniques:

- Friction to create heat to warm up the superficial tissue of the legs
- Compression to increase blood flow to the muscles of the legs and hips
- Shaking or rocking of the legs and hips to decrease excess tension

- Tapotement to stimulate the muscles of the legs and hip
- Range of motion of the legs and hips to decrease stiffness
- Gentle stretching to prepare muscles for the warm-up

While administering the preevent massage, the trainer should always be watching how the athlete is reacting to the preevent massage technique. The goal is always to have the athlete leave the table feeling prepared for athletic competition. Preevent massage is for stimulation and inspiration for the athlete. If the athlete is moving with ease and smiling, the trainer has done a great job.

DISCOVERY OF INJURIES

Occasionally when performing a preevent massage the trainer may notice that the athlete is in extreme pain or has an injury that may prevent her or him from competing safely. This situation is tricky because the trainer wants to have an open, trusting relationship with the athlete but does not want her or him to compete and experience further injury. Before starting to provide massages to athletes, the trainer should have in place a system of handling such situations.

Intake forms are part of the system to screen for pain and injuries before athletes receive a preevent massage. Watching how an athlete is moving before getting to the massage table can offer clues about possible trouble. Observing how the athlete is reacting to the preevent massage is crucial. The trainer should listen to the sounds that the athlete makes when receiving the preevent massage and question any unusual sounds or quick reactions.

Although a trainer does not have the authority to stop any athlete from competing, she can stop a treatment any time the treatment appears to be detrimental to the athlete. When working with a sports or medical team, a trainer should always consult with those who have higher authority when questions arise. The trainer should be prepared to explain to an athlete who is already in pain or injured before competing that the situation is likely to become worse. The trainer always wants to do what is best for the athlete.

CHAPTER 5

Postevent Massage Planning

The primary purpose of postevent massage is to assist the athlete in recovering from a workout or competition at an event site. After weeks and months of continuous workouts, the stress on the athlete's body can cause overtraining. Postevent massage between workouts can not only help the athlete's body recover but also create a psychological lift that may prevent burnout.

Postevent massage is never meant to interfere with an athlete's cool-down. The pace of the massage is much slower than that of preevent massage. The massage targets the muscles that the athlete has used in his sport. The emphasis should be placed on calming down the nervous system and flushing techniques to help the body return to homeostasis.

Postevent massage should start with light, slow, long gliding strokes that become heavier as the athlete's body adjusts to the pressure. Oil or lotion is applied as the gliding strokes are performed for ease of friction on skin. As the soreness decreases, petrissage, or kneading, strokes are applied to separate layers of tissue and flush metabolic waste products. Compression strokes follow to spread muscle fibers and restore blood flow to the muscles. Broadening strokes are then performed to lengthen and broaden sore, tight muscles. A return to long gliding strokes is done to soothe the muscles that have just been massaged. Gentle stretches are then applied to the muscles to enhance blood flow, restore length to the tissue, relieve soreness, and prevent postexercise joint stiffness.

POSTEVENT PRECAUTIONS

The trainer must have much more skill to perform postevent massage compared with preevent massage. After the athlete has completed her workout or competition, the trainer must determine whether the athlete is in a healthy enough state to receive postevent massage. At most triathlons and marathons a medical team is available to care for the athletes. Any sign that the athlete is in any physical difficulty should trigger a trip to the medical team. After the medical team has released the athlete and she has gone through a cool-down period, the trainer may then perform a postevent massage. An athlete should never be allowed to go straight from the activity to the massage table, especially at long-duration events.

Trainers must understand that their function at an event is to provide massage, not emergency medical services. But if no medical personnel are available in an emergency, a trainer may be required administer first aid until proper medical personnel arrive. The trainer providing the massages should have training in providing basic first aid skills. First aid and CPR training are not required to provide massage, but these skills can be useful at events.

Trainers providing postevent massage often encounter athletes suffering from dehydration, hyperthermia (too much heat building up in the body), and hypothermia (insufficient heat being produced by the body). Each of these conditions can become progressively worse, so the trainer needs to be able to spot the early signs of each. Generally, athletes who come for a postevent massage should be capable of responding to the trainer's questions about how they are feeling. They should not be too hot or too cold, and they should be able to get on and off a massage table without a great deal of difficulty.

LOGISTICAL AND RECORD-KEEPING PREPARATIONS

Postevent massage begins after the athletes have finished competing for the day. Whoever is coordinating the postevent massage must have a system for handling the athletes coming to receive massage. A sign-in sheet helps keep order at the massage site. Trainers simply massage the athletes in the order that they signed in. If the athletes will be filling out a postevent intake form, they can sign in and then fill out the intake form while they are waiting their turn to be massaged.

Most postevent massage intake forms include a full-body chart (see the form in chapter 1) so that the athletes can indicate which parts of the body need to be massaged. The trainer should look at how the body chart has been marked to determine whether the athlete will start faceup on the table or facedown. If the athlete marks the back of the legs, the athlete should start facedown. If the athlete marks both the front and the back of the legs, the athlete should start faceup on the table. In postevent massage, the trainer should monitor the physical condition of the athlete while administering the massage. Having the athlete lie in a face-up position when starting the postevent massage allows the trainer to communicate with the athlete more effectively and observe the athlete's facial expressions as the massage is being administered. Postevent massages should not be painful, so the trainer should watch for any signs that the massage is making the athlete uncomfortable.

IMPORTANCE OF THE COOL-DOWN

In horse racing the jockey never takes the winning horse directly from the finish line to the winner's circle. The horse always goes through a cool-down cycle. Taking a horse from a standing position to full exertion while running the race and then to a dead stop would be extremely stressful to the horse's body. The same is true for human athletes. Thus, all athletes should go through a proper cool-down cycle before receiving a postevent massage.

The physiological effects of a cool-down are just the opposite of the physiological effects of a warm-up. The body's heart rate, respiratory rate, and temperature should decrease gradually. Slow walking while drinking fluids is highly recommended. After the heart rate has slowed and body temperature has returned to normal, gentle stretches can be applied to maintain flexibility. Sometimes a proper cool-down is difficult to achieve when the weather is excessively hot or cold. Athletes need to be attired properly during cool-down. For this reason, trainers should make sure that athletes cannot go directly to the massage table after a workout or competition.

POSTEVENT MASSAGE INTERVIEW

Before the postevent massage begins, the trainer should watch the athlete approach the table, looking for any sign that the athlete is not walking normally or is in pain. If the athlete has completed a postevent intake form, the trainer should look at it before starting to interview the athlete. A short oral interview is done to make sure that the athlete can hear and respond to questions normally. The trainer should ask questions such as these: How are you today? What is bothering you the most? What part of your body would you like me to concentrate the postevent massage on?

The trainer should then advise the athlete about the correct position to take on the table. When beginning the massage, the trainer should say, "If anything I do makes you feel uncomfortable, please tell me." The trainer should let the athlete know that she is expected to give feedback as the massage is being administered. The athlete can tell the trainer whether the pressure of the massage is too deep or too light, whether the massage technique is painful, or which area of the body needs to be addressed. Communication between the athlete and the trainer is essential to an effective postevent massage.

SIMPLE INJURY RECOGNITION

Diagnosing injuries or prescribing treatments for injuries is not in the trainer's scope of practice, but any athlete who approaches a trainer for a postevent massage with unusual signs or symptoms should be evaluated before the massage begins. If during the premassage evaluation a trainer has concerns about the health of an athlete, the athlete should be referred to the proper medical personnel. Common injuries that athletes may have include superficial skin conditions (including inflammation, contusions, and lacerations), sprains, and strains.

- **Inflammation** is a local response to cellular injury. It may be identified by redness, heat, capillary dilation, and leukocyte infiltration. Leukocyte infiltration is the accumulation of cells in tissue not normal to the area. This condition is caused by damage to the tissue that then cannot maintain its proper structure. For example, capillaries, or small blood vessels, which are designed to deliver small amounts blood to healthy tissue, can be damaged by trauma that causes too much blood to enter an area of the body, resulting in a bruise. Inflammation is a normal response to injury repair and serves as a mechanism to eliminate painful agents and begin the repair process. During the inflammatory process, massage can be applied to decrease its severity.

- **Contusions** are injuries that occur to the tissues under the skin. Internal bleeding occurs without disruption of the epidermis or skin. When a muscle is damaged, tiny blood vessels are often broken, allowing blood to enter spaces where it is not ordinarily found, which causes contusions. Contusions are a problem because often they are not visible. Pressure from massage applied to the contusions is often painful. If contusions are massaged, bruising can occur and calcium can solidify, causing a hard calcium rock to form in muscle tissue. When contusions exist, massage is contraindicated in the area. The trainer can feel contusions by pressing on the area where they exist because they will have a spongy swollen feeling.

- **Lacerations** are breaks in the epidermis. Cuts or scrapes often occur during sporting activities when athletes fall or bang into each other or the ground. Massage should never be performed over open wounds. At bicycle races, athletes fall off their bicycles and suffer what is known as road rash. The superficial skin is scraped open. When this happens basic first aid should be applied to the area. Athletes who suffer from road rash have a difficult time lying on a massage table to receive a postevent massage.

- **Sprains and strains** are, after inflammation, contusions, and lacerations, the most common injuries likely to be encountered by athletes during workouts or at events. A sprain is an injury that occurs to a joint and, as you know from chapter 3, strains are injuries that occur in the muscle or tendon. Sprains and strains are not usually life threatening, but they can be extremely painful. Sprains and strains are classified as first degree, second degree, or third degree. A first-degree sprain or strain is the mildest. A third-degree strain or sprain is the most severe.

  Because sprain and strains are not life threatening, a trainer should be able to do simple joint and muscle tests to assess them. Muscle tests are performed by simply asking the athlete to contract a muscle against resistance. If the muscle has a strain, the athlete will feel discomfort right where the strain has occurred in the muscle. Joint tests are performed by stressing the joints in different directions. When conducting a simple joint test, the trainer usually stresses the joint to determine whether any ligament damage has occurred. When muscles are strained, the athlete will complain with joint movement. When joints are strained, the athlete will complain of joint instability. In mild cases of strains and sprains, athletes often continue playing or competing. As soon as possible after either strains or sprains occur, RICE should be applied.

FOCUS OF THE POSTEVENT MASSAGE

Runners and athletes who do a lot of running sometimes experience a runner's high, or a state of extreme euphoria. Endorphins are thought to act as natural painkillers, and the body produces them in greater quantities during exercise. These natural painkillers and the elevated temperature of the body make athletes a little numb. So immediately after they finish a workout or competition, they cannot feel their bodies as well as they can at other times. After athletes have had an opportunity to cool down and rest for a day, they are often much more aware of soreness in their bodies. For this reason, deep-tissue massage should not be administered during postevent massage. Athletes in this state are unable to give proper feedback to the trainer about the pressure being applied to them. The massage may feel OK at the moment but cause damage in the long run.

Research has shown the damage that exercise can cause in the muscles. Microtrauma occurs in the muscles. Actin filaments and myosin filaments are what we call the myofibrils of a muscle fiber. Actin and myosin filaments ratchet across each other as the muscle shortens. The actin and myosin filaments are attached to z-lines, and they pull the z-lines closer together as the muscle contracts (see figure 5.1). Photos taken of a marathon runner's muscles before a race show normal arrangement of actomyosin filaments and z-lines. Photos taken of the muscles after a race show the disruption of z-lines in muscle tissue because of damage from muscle contractions. The trainer treating the marathon runner in a postevent massage cannot see this tissue damage, but the athlete can definitely feel this microtrauma in postexercise soreness.

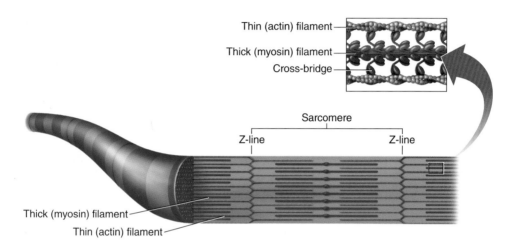

Figure 5.1 Actin and myosin filaments move past each other to create muscle contractions.

Given that athletes have completed their workouts or competition and may have some level of microscopic damage when they arrive for a postevent massage, the techniques used necessarily differ from those of the preevent massage. Postevent sport massage should never be painful! If an athlete has participated in a long-duration event, his body is likely to be slightly dehydrated and the muscles may be moderately inflamed. The postevent massage techniques are intended to help the athlete's body start to recover. Applying too much massage would be like putting the athlete's body through another workout.

A postevent massage should not last longer than 30 minutes when it is being administered immediately after an event. Additionally, postevent sport massage is often administered through clothing with oil applied only to the feet, legs, back, arms, and hands. The trainer wants to direct the postevent massage to the area of the body that most assists the athlete in recovery. For example, if the event required a lot of running the trainer would want to direct the postevent techniques to the legs and hips. The trainer might want to spend about 5 minutes doing postevent massage techniques on the front and back of each leg. The remaining 10 minutes could be used to massage any other area that the athlete would like the trainer to address.

Compressive effleurage is the first sport massage technique that should be applied in postevent massage to reduce soreness and inflammation. Compressive effleurage decreases excessive nerve stimulation in the area, increases localized circulation, which would bring healing new blood to the area, and assists in lymphatic drainage, which would encourage removal of fluid and metabolic waste product from the area. Compressive effleurage may be the most effective postevent massage technique that could be applied to speed the healing process of an athlete who participates in a long-duration event.

After compressive effleurage, the application of petrissage allows a smooth transition. As you learned in chapter 1, petrissage involves picking up and lifting muscle tissue while gently squeezing and kneading the muscle. When muscles become fatigued, they begin to spasm, which decreases their length and blood flow. This decrease in length and decrease in blood flow to the muscle can increase postexercise soreness. Petrissage applied with a comfortable amount of pressure eases painful stimulus to the sore muscle. The lifting and squeezing effect softens muscle tissue and assures that adhesions do not form within the muscle or from one muscle to another. The squeezing of the muscle tissue is also thought to create a milking action that aids in removal of metabolic waste from the tissue.

Following petrissage, compression technique is applied to the muscle bellies. Compression strokes are applied by applying pressure to the belly of a muscle with the palm of the hand. The palm is placed over the muscle, and pressure is added with a downward force, trapping the muscle belly between the palm of the hand and a bony surface of the body. When applying compression technique to the bellies of muscles that have been exhausted, great care must be taken to avoid applying too much pressure. Excessive pressure applied to a sore muscle belly can make the athlete extremely uncomfortable. The trainer must feel the resistance within the muscle belly with each downward movement. The application of compression technique to the belly of a muscle is thought to spread shortened muscle fibers. The fiber-spreading technique restores proper muscle tonus (continuous and passive partial contraction of the muscles), eases painful stimulus, and increases blood flow to the bellies of muscle. Compression strokes are essential to speed recovery in postevent massage.

A fourth technique, broadening strokes, may be applied as a smooth transition from compression strokes to a final round of compressive effleurage, which ends the postevent massage. Broadening strokes are applied with the palm of both hands centered on an extremity using increasing downward and outward pressure until the muscles under the hands are flattened and spread. This downward and outward movement is thought to increase the width of the muscles being treated, restoring the natural length to muscles that have shortened because of fatigue and postexercise soreness.

The finishing stroke for postevent massage should always be compressive effleurage. Compressive effleurage is a great technique to use at the end of a postevent treatment because it feels comforting and soothing. Remember that the purpose of compressive effleurage is to sedate overstimulated nerves, flush fluid, and restore blood flow to sore muscles that are in the cool-down process.

After the postevent massage is complete, stretching is administered to the massaged areas. Appropriate stretching can decrease muscle soreness, restore blood flow to the muscles, and increase pain-free range of motion. The postevent stretching should never be excessive because of the inflamed condition of the tissue and muscle soreness. The longer it takes to administer the postevent massage treatment, the more likely it is that the athlete's body temperature will drop. For that reason the postevent massage should not last longer than 30 minutes. When the athlete's body temperature drops during the cooling-down process, the athlete usually becomes a little stiff and movement is slightly more difficult. Stretching right after the postevent massage techniques have been administered helps reduce joint stiffness and may reduce postexercise soreness.

After the postevent massage has been completed, a brief interview should be conducted. This interview could be a simple as asking these questions: How are you feeling now? Did I cover the areas on your body that concerned you the most? The trainer should watch how the athlete is moving her or his body while getting up from the massage table. After lying on the table for 30 minutes, the athlete has to start the muscles actively working again. Sometimes the athlete will experience minor muscle spasms or cramps when getting off the table. The trainer should make sure that the athlete can stand up and walk without difficulty. The trainer can end a postevent massage treatment by saying to the athlete, "Thanks for letting me work with you. I hope what I have done has made you feel much better."

After the postevent massage the athlete should sense a feeling of recuperation, feel less muscle soreness, and have greater ease of movement. When you think of all the physiological changes that take place in the human body during exercise, undergoing a postevent massage makes a great deal of sense.

PART II

Applying Massage Techniques

CHAPTER 6

Stretching

The treatment for many low-back pain conditions used to be bed rest consisting of lying on the back with the knees bent, sometimes for weeks. This treatment protocol is no longer recommended because muscles become weaker and the joints become stiff with lack of use. In fact, the number one cause of decreased flexibility in muscles and joints is lack of use. The connective tissue or fascia of the muscle is usually what restricts muscle flexibility and joint range of motion. With inactivity, the fascial layers of the muscle can shorten, preventing muscles from functioning properly. Stretching can restore elasticity and flexibility to the connective tissue of the muscles to bring back proper function.

Other common causes of decreased flexibility are chronic tension, injuries, and disease, including arthritis. Chronic tension is excess tension that occurs in muscles for many reasons. Emotional upsets can increase muscular tension, and overuse or injury can create chronic tension. Chronic tension can cause muscles to become fibrotic and build up adhesions that restrict range of motion. Chronic tension can shorten muscle tissue and restrict joint capsule movement. Injury to a joint can cause damage to cartilage that blocks the joint from moving, and arthritic conditions can damage structure within the joint and make the joint painful to move. All of these should be considered before a vigorous stretching routine is established.

Additional causes for lack of flexibility include pain, trigger points, overuse syndromes, dehydration, poor nutrition, poor posture, poor circulation, stress, and infection. When pain signals are received in the brain from a muscle, the brain sends a motor response to tense the muscle, preventing movement and thereby decreasing its flexibility. Trigger points form in the muscle fibers, and they shorten the fibers and decrease the flexibility of the muscle. Overuse of a muscle increases irritation, which causes increased tension within it. Lack of fluid or dehydration can cause muscles to spasm or cramp, decreasing muscle flexibility. Poor nutrition affects the levels of ATP (muscle fuel), which allows the muscle fibers to release from contraction, decreasing flexibility. Poor posture creates differences in muscle lengths across joints, which decreases blood flow to muscles and limits their flexibility. Poor circulation decreases the flow of oxygen and nutrients to the muscles and reduces removal of metabolic waste, thus decreasing muscle flexibility. Stress triggers the fight or flight mechanism in the body, which increases muscular tension and decreases flexibility. Lastly, infection creates a toxic chemical imbalance in muscle tissue, which decreases muscle flexibility.

STRETCHING FUNDAMENTALS

As you learned in chapter 3, each muscle has three layers of connective tissue: epimysium, perimysium, and endomysium. After the layers of muscle, you come to the joint. The outer layer of a joint is called the joint capsule. Inside the joint capsule is a synovial membrane, a joint space, soft hyaline cartilage, and then bone. Ligaments attach the bones of the joint together and prevent unwanted movements of the joint. Any of these layers of tissue can restrict joint range of motion and decrease flexibility.

Now let's examine the basic terminology of stretching. *Stretching* is the movement of the body or its extremities to the full length or extent possible without causing damage to the tissue. Stretching is simply the elongation of tissue on one side of a joint. Each joint has a limit to how much the tissue crossing over it can be stretched without causing damage to the tissue. Care given to the amount of force applied during stretching is crucial to the effectiveness of the stretch.

Flexibility is the ability of muscles and joints to move through their full range of motion smoothly. All motions of the body require a certain amount of muscle and joint flexibility. Each joint has paired muscles that cross over the joint. All joints have natural muscles imbalances, meaning that muscles on one side of the joint are naturally stronger than muscles on the opposite side. The practice of daily stretching assures that these natural muscle imbalances across each joint stay within a healthy flexible margin.

The *range of motion* of a joint is the amount of movement that can occur at that specific location. Joint range of motion is measured by the extent of movement of a joint in degrees of a circle. A device called a goniometer, which is a circle with 360 degrees and two extending arms, is used to measure range of motion. One arm of the goniometer is fixed, and the other arm moves with the motion of the joint being measured. When the moveable arm stops at the limit of motion of the joint, the number of degrees between the arms can be read on the wheel between them.

The *anatomical range of motion* of a joint is the total possible range of motion of a joint. Without knowing the anatomical range of motion of a joint, it is impossible to know whether it has restrictions. If you ask an athlete to turn her head as far as possible, the chin should line up in a straight line with the shoulder. That movement is the anatomical range of motion of the neck. If the chin stops short of turning fully to the shoulder, an investigation about what structures are limiting the full rotation of the neck should occur.

Stretching muscles can be accomplished using a variety of techniques, including ballistic (bouncing), static (holding), tense relax (tensing a muscle and then stretching), or using reciprocal inhibition by contracting the opposite muscle that is to be lengthened. Many trainers use one or all of the techniques depending on the therapeutic outcome that they are trying to achieve. Let's take a closer look at each of these stretching techniques:

- **Ballistic stretching**, usually considered the least favored method of stretching, is accomplished by bouncing movements while joints are in the stretched position. The muscle and joint systems of the body have a protective mechanism built in that is called stretch reflex (also known as myotatic stretch reflex). When a joint goes through a range of motion, at some point the tissue being stretched starts to feel uncomfortable. That is a good thing. That uncomfortable feeling protects the muscle and joint from possible injury because generally a stretch that starts to feel uncomfortable is a warning not to add more pressure or hold in extended position for a long time. Muscles like to be stretched only so far and at a comfortable speed. Bouncing quickly engages the stretch reflex, which causes the muscle being stretched to contract. This action confuses the brain because it does not know whether the muscles involved are being stretched or contracted, and the bouncing motions can cause a muscle to snap back after being stretched, leading to muscle strains.

- **Static stretching** is accomplished by taking a joint through a range of motion and holding the joint in the stretched position for a period of seconds to minutes. This method of stretching is used often. Yoga stretching is an example of static stretching. A person moves into a yoga pose as far as he is comfortable and holds the pose while breathing and relaxing. Some people find this method of stretching to be spiritual and relaxing.

- **Tense relax stretching** is accomplished by taking a joint into a stretched position and then contracting the muscles being stretched for a period of seconds. The stretched muscles are relaxed for a few seconds, and then the joint is moved to a new position that continues to stretch the targeted muscles. The tense relax technique is useful in several situations.

An injured muscle is often unable to release completely. Using the tense relax method can help reeducate the muscle fibers by creating tension within the belly of the muscle and then releasing the tension to retrain it to elongate more efficiently.

• **Reciprocal inhibition** is accomplished by taking a joint into a stretched position and contracting the muscle opposing the one being stretched. All ranges of motion that a joint can accomplish have at least two muscles involved. When a joint goes through a range of motion, muscles on one side of the joint shorten and muscles on the other side of the joint must lengthen. When using the reciprocal inhibition technique, the opposing muscles are consciously contracted across the joint to increase the stretch on the side of the targeted muscles. Reciprocal inhibition can be used for reducing cramping in muscles. It is the natural process used when joints go through alternating ranges of motion.

BENEFITS OF STRETCHING

As the mind thinks, the body reacts. The number one reason to stretch is to keep a positive mental attitude. Most athletes deal with stress every day of their lives. The natural reaction to feeling stressed is to breathe shallowly and tense the body. The buildup of tension in the athletes' muscles creates greater resistance within the body. Reducing muscle tension increases the ease with which joints move through their full range of motion.

Healthy muscles must be elastic. They must stretch and contract efficiently. Engaging in a daily stretching routine helps decrease the effects of stress on the body and increases the likelihood that muscles will stay healthy. The healthier the muscles are, the quicker and more powerfully they can contract, which ultimately enhances the athlete's performance. Athletes who adopt a daily stretching routine will learn to enjoy stretching because they will feel better. When they feel the results, committing to a daily stretching routine becomes easier.

The application of stretching changes depending on its purpose. Preevent massage stretching is intended to assist warm-up; postevent stretching is intended to prevent excessive tension and postexercise soreness; and injury recovery stretching is intended to decrease muscle spasms, restore circulation, and reeducate the nervous system to the muscle. Preevent massage, designed to assist an athlete's warm-up, should always include therapeutic stretching. The warm-up increases the athlete's body temperature, which allows the muscles to stretch easier. Preevent massage and stretching reduces the chance that the athlete will incur an injury during competition. Postevent massage should also always include stretching because of postexercise muscle soreness. During exercise the buildup of lactic acid and other metabolic waste causes the muscles to become sore and stiffen. Stretching helps bring greater blood flow and oxygen to the muscles, enhancing the rejuvenation process.

When an athlete feels pain after an injury has occurred in his body, the brain automatically tightens that area of the body. The process is known as splinting. The brain does not like to feel pain, so it tries to limit movement in the area that is painful. Splinting decreases blood and oxygen flow and decreases range of motion to the area. Gentle stretching of areas of pain increases blood and oxygen flow, assisting in the healing process. In a rehabilitation setting, two of the most important goals are increasing range of motion and decreasing pain for the athlete. Athletes know immediately after treatment when they can move with less pain and whether their range of motion has improved to allow for normal movement at a joint. Those outcomes are what keep athletes coming back for treatments until they are no longer necessary.

Stretching also provides athletes with mental benefits and can improve longevity. When athletes stretch, they feel good and they enjoy their workouts more. When they are having fun, they usually compete at a more optimal level. Athletes who participate in a daily stretching routine enjoy a psychological advantage over those who do not. Older athletes usually lose a little speed and power as they age. Power is produced by the length of muscle fiber contraction and the number of fiber contracting. A regular stretching routine can maintain maximum muscle fiber length ratios. Those who engage in daily stretching routines enjoy a greater career span and maintain optimal performance levels throughout their careers.

Take a Deep Breath

Proper breathing is important to almost all functions of the human body. Bringing oxygen into the body as stretches are being performed helps the person who is stretching to relax. Tight muscles restrict the capillaries that deliver blood to the muscles. Breathing in brings in more oxygen to the lungs where it can be picked up by the blood and delivered to the muscles.

Learning to breathe in a deep relaxed way while stretching takes a great deal of concentration, especially in the beginning. Most people have a tendency to hold their breath as they feel a joint go through a range of motion and the muscles begin to stretch. The usual reaction of the athlete being stretched is to anticipate the stretch sensation and guard against further overstretching by holding his breath and tensing the muscle being stretched. A much more effective approach is to inhale first and then exhale when going through a range of motion as the muscles begin to stretch. Athletes must learn how to let go so that their muscles can stretch effectively.

CONSISTENT PRACTICE

Muscle contraction and muscle inhibition is a cooperative function of the nervous system and the muscular system. The law of facilitation states that after a stimulus passes through a certain set of neurons to the exclusion of others, the following stimulus will continue to take the same pathway. The more often the stimulus takes the pathway, the less resistance it experiences. This relationship is referred to in the adage "Practice makes perfect." Any behavior, bad or good, repeated enough times will become easier and easier to do, so learning to stretch correctly takes practice. The more often the correct method of stretching is practiced, the smaller becomes the resistance to the effectiveness of the stretch.

Increasing and maintaining all ranges of motion of all the joints in the body is the goal of a good flexibility routine. To maintain full range of motion of all the joints in the body, athletes need a systematic method of moving each joint through every range of motion for that joint. Then, they need to repeat the motions numerous times while concentrating on breathing and letting go at the same time. The more they practice the system, the easier it becomes. Superior flexibility is achieved only by a commitment to daily practice.

Many athletes are extremely flexible in certain ranges of motion of certain joints in their bodies but are not flexible in other ranges of motions in other joints. The tendency with most athletes is to repeat the ranges of motion that they are good at and avoid the others. Smart athletes choose to find the ranges of motion in which they do not do well and practice repetitions of them until they master the difficult ones.

ACTIVE ISOLATED STRETCHING

Before athletes begin stretching, they should engage in warm-up activities. Remember that the purpose of a warm-up is to elevate body temperature, increase respiratory rate, increase circulation, and prepare the neural pathways. Riding a stationary bike until perspiration begins (usually about 10 minutes) is an effective way to warm up.

Three main concepts are important to the application of active isolated stretching: identify, isolate, and intensify. The first step in effective stretching is to identify the muscles that are to be stretched. The second step is to put the athlete in the proper position to isolate the muscles targeted to stretch. The third step is to intensify the activity necessary to achieve the optimal stretch of the muscles targeted.

Athletes can perform any of the stretches in this chapter (starting on page 74) by themselves. Each stretch provides the information needed for athletes to perform the stretches correctly on their own. But a trainer or another athlete serving as a stretch partner can provide assistance during any or all of these stretches. Assisted stretching works well because another person can watch the athlete's body position and add a little extra stretch at the end of most ranges of motion. The athlete and the person assisting must communicate well. The timing of the movements and the amount of force used must be appropriate. Athletes and trainers must remember that muscles are most vulnerable to injury at the very end of a stretch.

As an example of stretching with assistance, let's use the straight leg raise to review the steps of active isolated stretching. The straight leg raise is performed by lying faceup and raising a leg toward the head while keeping the knee locked. Step one of active isolated stretching is to identify the muscles to be stretched. The straight leg raise stretches the hamstrings. The second step is to position the athlete in the most effective position to stretch the targeted muscles. For the hamstrings, this is lying faceup. Muscles should never be stretched in the weight-bearing position because they cannot stretch and contract at the same time. The athlete should breathe out while performing the stretch. The athlete should not overcontract the quadriceps muscles to keep the knee locked nor force the leg forward with too much effort to stretch the hamstrings. An effort that is so intense that it causes the athlete to strain defeats the purpose of the stretch.

The third step is to intensify the activity to achieve the optimal stretch. The trainer or stretching partner should guide the athlete's hip joint though the range of motion and add about 2 pounds (1 kg) of pressure at the end of the range of motion. The trainer takes the athlete's joint through a range of motion that stretches the muscle only to the soft end feel, which occurs at the end of range of motion where the muscle feels as if it still has room to stretch. At this point, the athlete should be breathing out. A muscle should never be forced to stretch.

The hamstrings should be held in the stretched position for no more than two seconds. Then the trainer or partner assists the athlete in returning the leg to the resting position on the massage table. While the leg is in the resting position, the athlete should breathe in while the trainer shakes the just stretched leg to make sure that the athlete is not holding tension in the leg. Shaking works well in the arms and legs to remind the athlete to let go of tension and relax the muscles being stretched between repetitions. The straight leg stretch should be performed for 8 to 10 repetitions. Athletes in good physical condition can do three sets (8 to 10 repetitions each) of stretches for each group of muscles.

For the most effective stretching routine, every range of motion of every joint in the body should be stretched as often as necessary to maintain full range of motion. Muscles in which the athlete needs better flexibility should be targeted. Muscles should never be overstretched, particularly recently injured muscles. The trainer or partner should always observe the athlete's reaction to the stretching application. If the process becomes painful, stretching should be discontinued and application reassessed.

NECK STRETCHES

To stretch the neck, the athlete starts in a standing position and leans forward with the knees slightly bent and the hands on the knees for support. To warm up the neck, the athlete circumducts the neck by moving the head around in circles, performing 8 to 10 circles in each direction.

Cervical Flexion

The athlete tucks the chin and tries to touch it to the chest. He places the hands behind the head and contracts the muscles in the front of the neck to bring the chin toward the chest. Then the athlete gently pulls with the hands on the back of the head to increase the range of motion. He holds the stretched position for two seconds and then lifts the chin until he is looking straight ahead. The athlete should complete 8 to 10 repetitions.

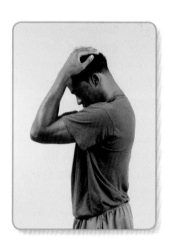

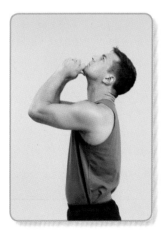

Cervical Extension

The athlete places the hands under the chin and contracts the muscles on the back of the neck so that the head moves to look up at the ceiling. He gently pushes up with the hands to increase the range of motion, holds for two seconds, and then returns the head to a straightforward-looking position. If this stretch causes pain or discomfort, it should not be continued. The athlete should perform 8 to 10 repetitions.

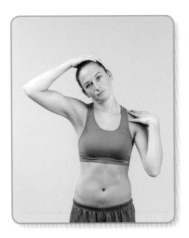

Lateral Flexion

The athlete attempts to touch the ear to the same-side shoulder. Placing the same-side hand on the top (opposite side) of the head helps to extend the stretch. Contracting the muscles on the side of the neck brings the ear toward the shoulder. The athlete holds the stretch for two seconds and then returns the head to the straight-up position. She completes 8 to 10 stretches on one side and then performs the stretch 8 to 10 times on the opposite side.

Cervical Rotation

The athlete turns the chin to one shoulder, places the same-side hand on the chin, places the opposite hand on the back of the head, and uses both hands to assist rotation of the neck to that side. He holds the stretch for two seconds and then returns the head to the straightforward position. The athlete performs the stretch 8 to 10 times on that side and then performs the stretch 8 to 10 times on the opposite side.

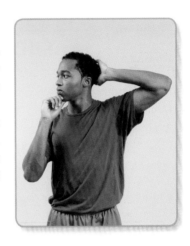

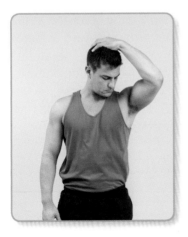

Cervical Flexion With 45-Degree Head Turn

The athlete turns the head 45 degrees to one side and uses the muscles on the front of the neck to bring the neck into flexion. He places one hand on the top and back of the head, gently pulls the neck toward the chest for two seconds, and then returns to the straightforward position. The athlete does 8 to 10 repetitions on that side and then performs the stretch 8 to 10 times on the opposite side.

Cervical Hyperextension With 45-Degree Head Turn

The athlete places the hand on the side of the neck to be stretched under the chin. She turns the head to a 45-degree angle, extends the neck backward to the side, holds for two seconds, and then returns the head to the straightforward position. The athlete does 8 to 10 repetitions on that side and then performs the stretch 8 to 10 times on the opposite side.

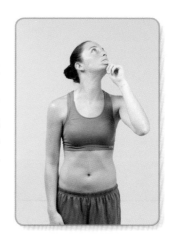

SHOULDER STRETCHES

To warm up the shoulders, the athlete starts in a standing position and leans forward with the knees slightly bent. He performs circumduction of the shoulders by bending forward and gently making circles with the arms, doing 8 to 10 circles in alternating directions.

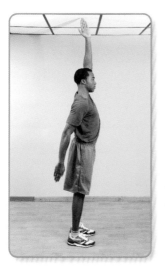

Opposite Arm Flexion and Extension Stretch

The athlete stands with the arms hanging down at the sides. Without bending the elbows, he brings one arm forward straight above the head and at the same time brings the other arm backward as far as it moves in that direction comfortably. The athlete holds each arm in the stretched position for two seconds, brings the arms down to the sides, moves the arms in the opposite direction, and holds for two seconds. He repeats the stretch 8 to 10 times in both directions.

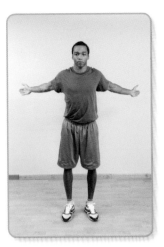

Chest Stretch With Arms Extended

The athlete starts in a standing position with the arms extended at shoulder level in front and the palms together. While keeping the arms straight, he moves the hands as far apart as possible while contracting the midback muscles, holds the stretched position for two seconds, and then returns the arms to the starting position. The athlete performs 8 to 10 repetitions.

Chest Stretch With Arms Extended 45 Degrees Above Shoulders

The athlete stands with the arms extended 45 degrees above shoulder level and the palms together. She brings the arms as far apart as possible while contracting the posterior upper shoulder muscles, holds in stretched position for two seconds, and then returns the arms to the front of the body. The athlete performs 8 to 10 repetitions.

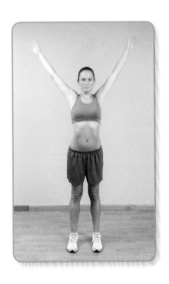

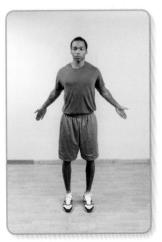

Chest Stretch With Arms Extended 45 Degrees Below Shoulders

The athlete stands with the arms extended 45 degrees below shoulder level and the palms together. He bring the arms as far apart as possible while contracting the posterior lower shoulder muscles, holds in stretched position for two seconds, and then returns the arms to the front of the body. The athlete performs 8 to 10 repetitions.

Arm Extension Stretch

The athlete stands with the arms by the sides. He moves the arms back behind the body as far as possible without bending the elbows and holds in stretched position for two seconds. The athlete performs 8 to 10 repetitions.

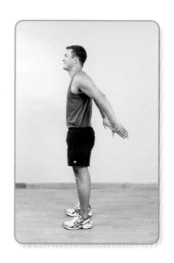

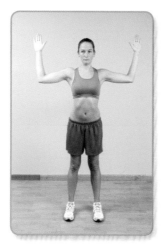

Medial Rotator Shoulder Stretch

The athlete stands with both arms in front at shoulder height. She bends the elbows 90 degrees with the palms facing forward, rotates the shoulders externally as far as possible, and holds for two seconds. The athlete performs 8 to 10 repetitions.

Lateral Rotator Shoulder Stretch

The athlete stands with both arms in front at shoulder height. He bends the elbows 90 degrees with the palms facing backward, rotates the shoulders internally as far as possible, and holds for two seconds. The athlete performs 8 to 10 repetitions.

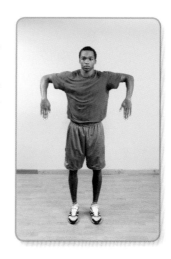

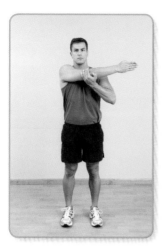

Posterior Shoulder Stretch

The athlete stands with one arm in front at shoulder height and moves that arm straight across the front of the body, pressing the arm into the chest. The other hand assists the stretch by pushing at the back of the elbow. The shoulders should be kept level from one side to the other through the entire stretch. The stretch is held for two seconds. The athlete performs the stretch 8 to 10 times on one side and then performs the stretch 8 to 10 times on the opposite side.

Side Shoulder Stretch

From a standing position, the athlete brings one arm from the side of the body straight over the shoulder behind the head as far as possible, assisting the stretch by pulling on the elbow with the opposite hand. After holding the stretch for two seconds, she returns the arm to the side. The athlete performs the stretch 8 to 10 times on one arm and then performs the stretch 8 to 10 times on the opposite arm.

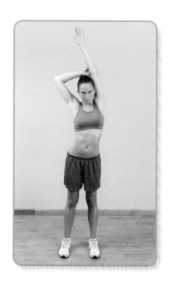

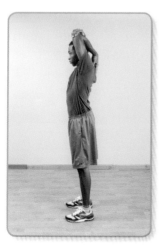

Triceps Shoulder Stretch

The athlete stands with one arm raised to shoulder height and the palm facing up. He flexes the elbow until the hand is resting on the shoulder with the elbow pointing straight forward. With the opposite hand, the athlete gently lifts the elbow up and straight back as far as possible and holds for two seconds. He completes 8 to 10 stretches with one arm and then 8 to 10 stretches with the opposite arm.

Posterior Hand Touch

The athlete stands with one arm straight over the shoulder, bends the elbow behind the head with the palm facing the body, and reaches down. He moves the opposite arm behind the back with the elbow bent and the palm facing out, reaches up with that hand, and tries to touch the hands behind the back. If the athlete is flexible enough, the hands can join at the fingers. The athlete completes this stretch 8 to 10 times, switches arm positions, and completes 8 to 10 stretches on the opposite side.

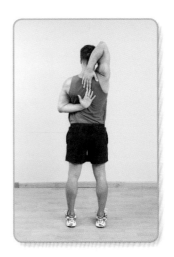

WRIST AND ELBOW STRETCHES

Many sports stress the wrists and elbows through throwing a ball or swinging a club or racquet. Stretching the wrists can relieve some of the soreness and tightening of the forearm muscles. Golfer's elbow and tennis elbow are common overuse syndromes of the forearm muscles that respond well to stretching after the acute stage of injury has passed.

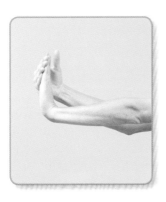

Wrist Flexor Stretch

The athlete extends one arm in front at shoulder height with the palm facing down and the fingers straight. She bends one wrist up and back, assisting the stretch by using the other hand to pull the fingers gently back, and holds the fingers and wrist in the stretched position for two seconds before returning the wrist to palm-down position. The athlete completes 8 to 10 stretches with one arm and then completes 8 to 10 stretches with the other arm.

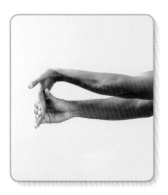

Wrist Extensor Stretch

The athlete extends one arm in front at shoulder height with the palm facing up and the fingers straight. He bends the wrist up and back, assisting the stretch by using the opposite hand to help pull the fingers back, and holds the fingers and wrist in stretched position for two seconds before returning the wrist to palm-up position. The athlete completes 8 to 10 stretches with one arm and then completes 8 to 10 stretches with the other arm.

Wrist Adductor Stretch

The athlete bends one elbows to 90 degrees with the palm facing inward. Using the other hand, he moves the wrist upward away from the forearm until the wrist stops. The athlete should hold the stretch for two seconds before returning to the starting position. The athlete completes 8 to 10 stretches with one wrist and then completes 8 to 10 stretches with the other wrist.

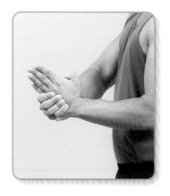

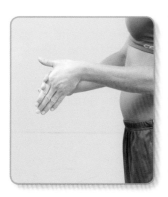

Wrist Abductor Stretch

The athlete bends one elbow to 90 degrees with the palm facing inward. Using the other hand, she moves the wrist downward away from the forearm until the wrist stops. The athlete should hold the stretch for two seconds before returning to the starting position. The athlete completes 8 to 10 stretches with one wrist and then completes 8 to 10 stretches with the other wrist.

Wrist Supinator Stretch

The athlete starts with one arm at the side with the elbow bent to 90 degrees and the palm facing up. With the fingers of the opposite hand, he reaches under the hand that is being stretched, grabs the thumb side of the hand, twists the wrist away from the body, and holds for two seconds. The athlete completes 8 to 10 stretches on one hand and repeats the stretch 8 to 10 times on the other hand.

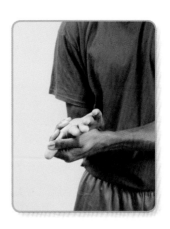

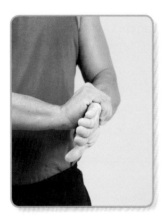

Wrist Pronator Stretch

The athlete starts with one arm at the side with the elbow bent to 90 degrees and the palm facing down. With the fingers of the opposite hand, he reaches across the hand that is being stretched, grabs the bottom of the little finger side, twists the wrist toward the body, and holds for two seconds. The athlete completes 8 to 10 stretches on one hand and repeats the stretch 8 to 10 times on the other hand.

BACK STRETCHES

One of the most common complaints of athletes is low-back pain. Tight muscles in the low back force the athlete to compensate by overusing the legs and arm muscles. Stretching the low-back muscles protects the back and prevents injuries that can occur when other muscles in the body must compensate for the back muscles.

Single-Leg Knee to Chest

The athlete lies faceup on the floor and brings one knee up toward the chest as far as is comfortable. He places both hands on top of the knee, pulls it into the chest, and holds for two seconds. The athlete completes 8 to 10 stretches on one leg and repeats the stretch 8 to 10 times on the other leg.

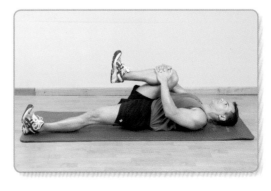

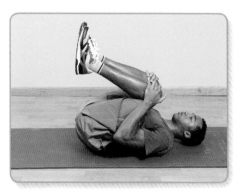

Double-Leg Knee to Chest

The athlete lies faceup on the floor and brings both legs up toward his chest as far as is comfortable. With a hand on top of each knee, he pulls the knees into the chest and holds for two seconds. The athlete completes 8 to 10 stretches.

Bent-Knee Trunk Flexion Stretch

The athlete sits on the edge of a chair with the feet on the floor and the legs about shoulder-width apart. He leans forward, places the hands on top of the feet, drops the head between the legs as far as is comfortable, holds for two seconds, and then returns to the sitting position. The athlete completes 8 to 10 stretches.

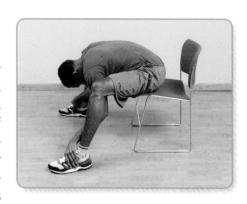

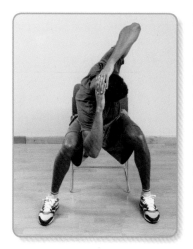

Upper Trunk Rotation Stretch

From a seated position on the edge of a chair, the athlete spreads the legs about shoulder-width apart and places the hands behind the head. He twists the trunk, leans forward, drops the head between the legs as far as is comfortable, holds for two seconds, and then returns to the sitting position. The athlete performs 8 to 10 repetitions and then switches to perform the stretch 8 to 10 times on the opposite side.

Lateral Trunk Side-Bending Stretch

From a standing position, the athlete slides one hand down the side of the leg as far as possible, brings the opposite arm up over the head, holds for two seconds, and returns to the standing position. She performs 8 to 10 repetitions and then switches to perform the stretch 8 to 10 times on the opposite side.

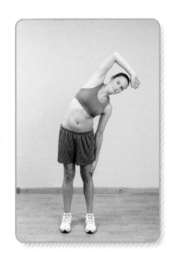

HIP AND KNEE STRETCHES

The knee is the most complex joint in the body. It must flex, extend, and rotate without restrictions in any sport that requires running. Restrictions in the hip muscles can affect the knees. Stretching the muscles surrounding the hips and knees helps prevent injuries.

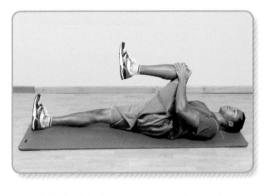

Gluteus Maximus Stretch

While lying on the back with one leg straight on the floor, the athlete raises the other thigh to 90 degrees and flexes the knee to 90 degrees. The thigh will be perpendicular to the floor, and the lower leg will be parallel to the floor. He pulls the bent knee in the direction of the opposite shoulder as far as is comfortable, holds for two seconds, and returns to the starting position. The athlete performs 8 to 10 repetitions and then switches legs to perform the stretch 8 to 10 times on the opposite side.

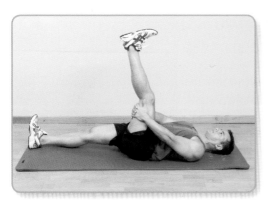

Bent-Knee Hamstring Stretch

Lying on the floor in the face-up position with one leg flat on the ground, the athlete raises the other thigh to 90 degrees and flexes the knee to 90 degrees. The thigh will be perpendicular to the floor, and the lower leg will be parallel to the floor. Holding below the knee with both hands, he straightens the knee as far as is comfortable, holds for two seconds, and returns to the starting position. The athlete performs 8 to 10 repetitions and then switches legs to perform the stretch 8 to 10 times on the opposite side.

Straight-Leg Hamstring Stretch

Lying on the floor in the face-up position with one leg flat on the ground, the athlete raises the other leg as far as is comfortable without letting the knee bend, holds below the knee with both hands for two seconds, and returns to the starting position. She performs 8 to 10 repetitions and then switches legs to perform the stretch 8 to 10 times on the opposite side.

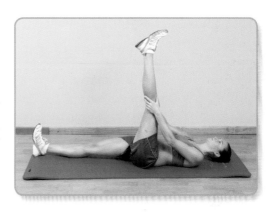

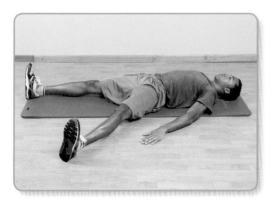

Adductor Groin Stretch

Lying on the floor in the face-up position with the legs together, the athlete brings one leg out to the side as far as is comfortable, holds for two seconds, and then returns to the starting position. He performs 8 to 10 repetitions and then switches legs to perform the stretch 8 to 10 times on the opposite side.

Figure-Four Iliotibial Band Stretch

Lying on the floor in the face-up position with the legs together, the athlete brings one leg straight up into a 90-degree position and then crosses the leg over the front of the body as far as is comfortable. He tries to keep the hips flat on the floor, assisting the crossing leg with the same-side arm, if necessary, and then returns to the starting position. The athlete performs 8 to 10 repetitions and then switches legs to perform the stretch 8 to 10 times on the opposite side.

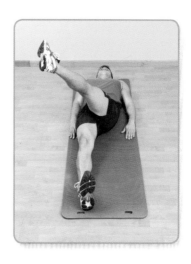

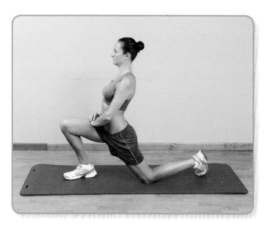

Hip Flexor Psoas Stretch

From a kneeling position, the athlete brings one knee forward with the foot on the floor, drops the other leg straight behind the trunk, leans backward as far as is comfortable with the hands on the thigh for support, holds for two seconds, and then returns to the starting position. The athlete performs 8 to 10 repetitions and then switches legs to perform the stretch 8 to 10 times on the opposite side.

Side-Lying Quadriceps Stretch

Lying on the side, the athlete brings the bottom knee toward the chest to 90 degrees. He holds the opposite ankle, brings the upside knee back in a straight line until it is even with the trunk, holds for two seconds, and then returns to the starting position. The athlete performs 8 to 10 repetitions and then switches legs to perform the stretch 8 to 10 times on the opposite side.

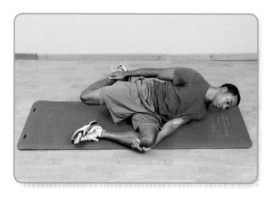

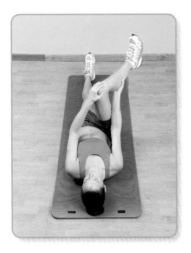

Internal Hip Rotation Stretch

While lying on the back with one leg straight on the floor, the athlete raises the other thigh to 90 degrees and flexes the knee to 90 degrees. The thigh will be perpendicular to the floor, and the lower leg will be parallel to the floor. She rotates the leg as far as is comfortable away from the center of the body with one hand on the knee and the other hand gently rotating the leg in an outward direction by pulling on the calf. The athlete holds for two seconds and then returns to the starting position. She performs 8 to 10 repetitions and then switches legs to perform the stretch 8 to 10 times on the opposite side.

External Hip Rotation Stretch

While lying on the back with one leg straight on the floor, the athlete raises the other thigh to 90 degrees and flexes the knee to 90 degrees. The thigh will be perpendicular to the floor, and the lower leg will be parallel to the floor. He rotates the leg toward the center of the body with one hand on the knee and the other hand gently rotating the leg in an inward direction by pulling on the ankle as far as is comfortable. The athlete holds for two seconds then returns to the starting position. He performs 8 to 10 repetitions and then switches legs to perform the stretch 8 to 10 times on the opposite side.

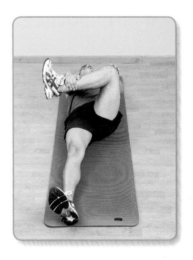

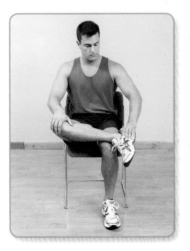

Knee Internal Rotation Stretch

While sitting in a chair, the athlete crosses one leg over the other so that the foot is past the top of the leg. He turns the foot on the crossed-over leg downward toward the floor as far as is comfortable, assisting with the hand, holds for two seconds, and returns to the starting position. The athlete performs 8 to 10 repetitions and then switches legs to perform the stretch 8 to 10 times on the opposite side.

Knee External Rotation Stretch

While sitting in a chair, the athlete crosses one leg over the other so that the foot is past the opposite leg. He turns the foot on the crossed-over leg upward toward the ceiling as far as is comfortable, assisting with the hand, holds for two seconds, and returns to the starting position. The athlete performs 8 to 10 repetitions and then switches legs to perform the stretch 8 to 10 times on the opposite side.

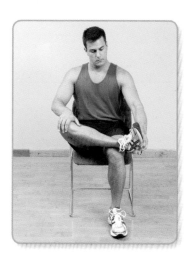

ANKLE AND CALF STRETCHES

One of the most common injuries in sports is spraining the ankle. Overuse of lower leg muscles and tightening of the ankle joint itself increases the possibility of injury to the ankle. One of the best methods for preventing injuries to the ankle is to maximize the amount of flexibility at the ankle joint.

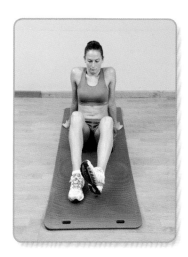

Circumduction of Ankle

While sitting on the floor, the athlete points the foot and moves it in circular rotations in both directions 10 to 12 times. She then switches legs to perform the movement with the opposite ankle.

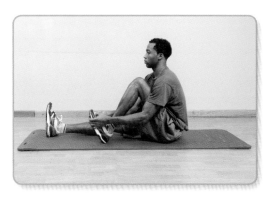

Deep Calf Stretch for Soleus

While sitting on the floor with one knee bent, the athlete flexes the foot on the bent leg toward the shin on the same leg, assisting the movement with the hands, holds for two seconds, and returns to the starting position. He performs 8 to 10 repetitions and then switches feet to perform 8 to 10 repetitions on the opposite foot.

Achilles Tendon Stretch

While sitting on the floor with one knee bent, the athlete brings the foot on the bent leg as close to the butt as possible. She flexes the foot on the bent leg toward the shin, assisting with the hands, holds for two seconds, and returns to the starting position. She performs 8 to 10 repetitions and then switches feet to perform 8 to 10 repetitions on the opposite foot.

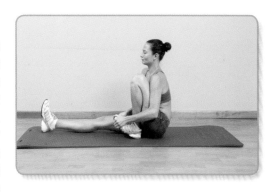

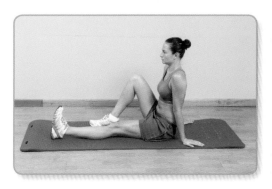

Superficial Calf Stretch for Gastrocnemius

While sitting on the floor with one knee bent and the opposite leg straight, the athlete flexes the foot on the straight leg toward the shin, holds for two seconds, and returns to the starting position. She performs 8 to 10 repetitions and then switches feet to perform 8 to 10 repetitions on the opposite foot.

Inversion Ankle Stretch

While sitting on the floor with one knee bent and the opposite leg straight, the athlete turns the foot on the straight leg inward, holds for two seconds, and returns to the starting position. He performs 8 to 10 repetitions and then switches feet to perform 8 to 10 repetitions on the opposite foot.

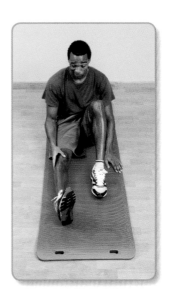

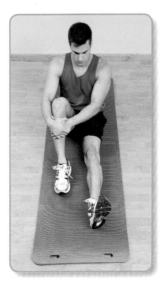

Eversion Ankle Stretch

While sitting on the floor with one knee bent and the opposite leg straight, the athlete turns the foot on the straight leg outward, holds for two seconds, and returns to the starting position. He performs 8 to 10 repetitions and then switches feet to perform 8 to 10 repetitions on the opposite foot.

CHAPTER 7

Pre- and Postevent Massage

In this chapter, the techniques for pre- and postevent massage will be reviewed and then suggested routines are offered for pre- and postevent massage. The massage routines are divided into upper-body and lower-body routines. At some events not enough time is available to apply massage to the entire body of the athlete. By dividing the routines into the upper body and lower body, the trainer can decide which is more important for the sport and the athlete. If performing both upper- and lower-body routines, the trainer should alter the order of the routines to finish massaging the front or back of the athlete before having her or him turn over to the other side of the body.

Recommendations are offered for how long the strokes should be applied and how many times the strokes should be repeated during the massage routines. Most pre- and postevent sport massage is applied quickly because of the limited time available and the number of athletes that the trainer must massage at an event. Trainers should feel free to experiment with what works best for them.

PREEVENT SPORT MASSAGE

Remember from chapter 4 that the purpose of a preevent sport massage is to help prepare the athlete for a workout or competition, to assist the athlete in warming up, to increase circulation to the muscles, to maintain the athlete's flexibility, to prevent injury, and to provide a psychological lift before a workout or competition. Athletes often ask for minor assistance such as stretching the hamstrings or massaging the neck. They are not looking for a full-body massage or even an upper- or lower-body preevent routine. Athletes can be superstitious and nervous just before competition. The trainer needs to provide the type of treatment that reduces the athlete's preevent nervousness but does not get in the way of the athlete's precompetition preparation. The following massage routine can be applied to achieve the desired intent for preevent sport massage.

Circular Friction

Circular friction is applied with hand-over-hand movements in circular motions to warm up tissue and increase blood supply to skin and underlying tissue. Circular friction is applied to the shoulder and back from the shoulder down the back from the opposite side of the table that the trainer is standing on. The trainer should apply enough pressure to move the skin under the hands in circular motions. The skin must not be stuck to the muscles directly beneath it and must be able to move freely in all directions.

Friction

Friction in preevent sport massage can be applied by rapid movement of the hands in a back-and-forth motion with superficial contact. This technique rapidly creates warmth to assist the warm-up. Back-and-forth friction techniques can be used to target the extremities. Friction is great for warming up smaller areas of the body like the forearm and upper arm or the calf and thigh before moving to techniques that target deeper tissue. Rapid friction is accomplished by moving both hands back and forth over a specific area. The movement is done quickly and takes only a few seconds to do over each part of the body. Its major purpose is to create heat over small parts of the body quickly. Rapid friction is used on the arms and legs.

Jostling and Shaking

Jostling and shaking is performed by lifting or shaking a part of the athlete's body rapidly. It is applied to the athlete to stimulate the nervous system, usually toward the end of the massage.

Tapotement

Tapotement is performed by rapid movements of the hands striking the athlete's body with various levels of pressure depending on what part of the body tapotement is applied to. Tapotement includes beating, tapping, hacking, slapping, and cupping. The type of tapotement also changes depending on the part of the body it is applied to.

Compression

Compression is applied by a rhythmic pressing of the deeper tissue. Whereas friction is applied to warm up superficial tissue, compression is applied to increase blood flow to the deeper tissue that it is applied to.

Range of Motion

Range of motion of joints is accomplished by simply moving the joint through motions that will be required by the athlete to compete or work out. The trainer often does range of motion passively. Range of motion is performed to stimulate synovial fluid, which lubricates the athlete's joints. Range of motion also prepares the athlete's joints for therapeutic stretching.

Therapeutic Stretching

Therapeutic stretching is performed by moving an athlete's joint through a range of motion until resistance is felt. Some types of stretching involve holding the athlete in the stretched position for many seconds, whereas other types require holding in the stretched position for only two seconds. The two-second hold method of stretching is usually applied six or eight times. The purpose of therapeutic stretching is to assist the warm-up, bring blood flow to the stretched muscles, release excess tension, and prevent injuries. (Refer to chapter 6 for more information on stretching.)

ADMINISTERING A PREEVENT MASSAGE

A preevent sport massage will probably be administered with the athlete wearing clothing. As noted in chapter 4, oils or lubricants are usually not used because they can clog the pores in the skin or give an athlete an unfair advantage in some events. The preevent massage should not last longer than 10 to 15 minutes because the trainer does not want to relax the athlete so much that lethargy ensues. Upbeat music can be played during the massage, and the trainer should use inspiring conversation while administering the massage.

Upper-body preevent massage is designed to target the muscles of the upper body. The trainer often does not have enough time to apply preevent massage to the athlete's entire body. Sports like baseball, tennis, and golf require a lot of upper-body movement, so targeting the upper body with preevent massage helps prevent unnecessary injuries and allows the athlete to prepare for fast upper-body movement. Lower-body massage targets the muscles of the lower body and is likely to be the area treated in preevent massage for athletes who participate in running or sports that require a lot of running.

UPPER-BODY PREEVENT ROUTINE

Posterior Upper Body

The trainer starts with the athlete lying facedown because the larger and bulkier muscles of the upper body are on the back of the body. Targeting those muscles first helps the athlete relax and decreases excess tension in the shoulder and back. The trainer starts with the back and shoulder on one side of the body and then works on the arm on that side. When that is complete, the trainer repeats steps 1 through 10 on the other side of the athlete's body.

1. Apply circular friction to the back and shoulder of the athlete.

2. Apply compression strokes three times next to the spine up the back.

3. Gently squeeze the area between the shoulders and neck.

4. Apply friction to the forearm from the wrist to the elbow, using brisk back-and-forth motions with both hands.

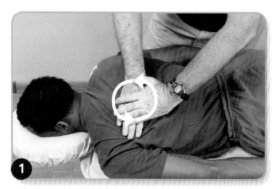

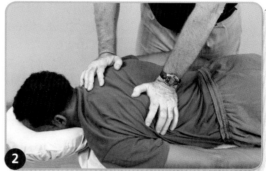

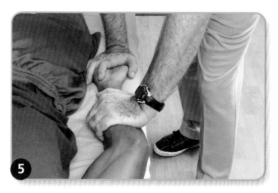

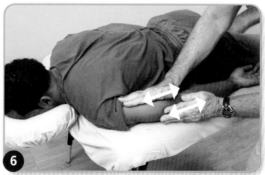

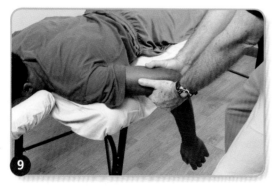

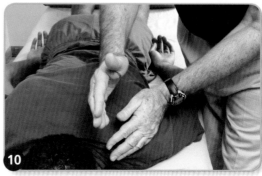

5. Apply compression strokes to the forearm from the elbow to the wrist three times.

6. Apply friction to the back of the upper arm from the shoulder to the elbow, using brisk back-and-forth motions with both hands.

7. Apply compression to the back of the upper arm from the shoulder to the elbow three times.

8. Apply range of motion and lift and drop the scapula. Place one hand under the anterior shoulder at the deltoid muscle, gently lift the shoulder off the table, and then let it drop back on to the table. When lifting the shoulder and letting it go, the trainer wants the shoulder to flop back to the table. This action helps the athlete let go of tension in the shoulder. Apply three to four times.

9. Apply range of motion to the arm by putting the hands under the athlete's upper arm and gently rocking the upper arm back and forth in internal and external rotation.

10. Apply tapotement to the shoulder and back, starting at the shoulder and working down the back.

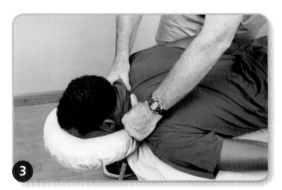
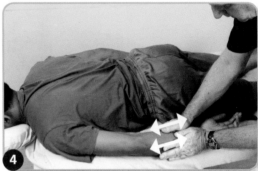
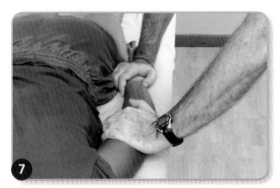
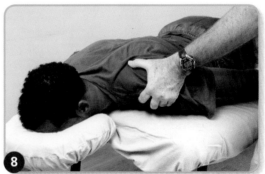

Anterior Upper Body

Now the trainer is ready to apply preevent massage to the front of the body. The athlete moves to the face-up position for the second part of the preevent upper-body massage. Remember that part of the purpose of preevent massage is to inspire the athlete just before competition. With the athlete in the face-up position the trainer can look the athlete in the eye while talking. The trainer performs steps 1 through 10 on one side of the athlete's body and then repeats the process on the other side.

1. Apply friction to one forearm using brisk back-and-forth motions with both hands from the wrist to the elbow for 10 seconds.
2. Apply compression strokes to the forearm from the elbow to the wrist three times.
3. Apply friction strokes to the upper arm using brisk back-and-forth motions with both hands from the shoulder to the elbow for 10 seconds.
4. Apply compression strokes to the upper arm from the shoulder to the elbow three times.

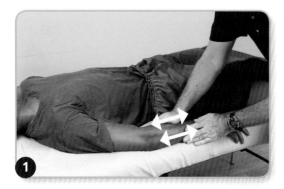
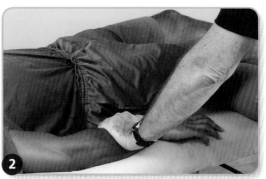
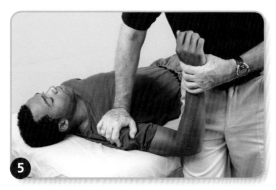
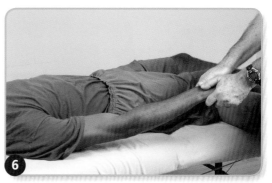
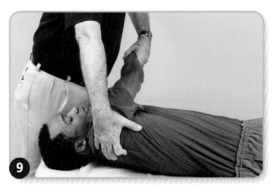
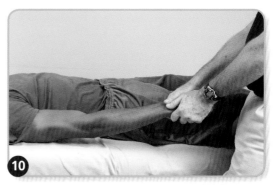

5. Apply compression strokes to the chest, upper arm, and forearm three times.

6. Apply a gentle stretch of the arm downward toward the feet. Hold the athlete's hand with both hands and gently pull the arm toward the athlete's feet.

7. Apply a gentle stretch of the arm outward away from the body. Hold the athlete's hand with both hands, bring the athlete's arm out straight to shoulder height, and then gently pull the athlete's arm away from the body.

8. Apply a gentle stretch of the arm overhead. Hold the athlete's hand with both hands, bring the athlete's arm up straight over the head, and gently stretch.

9. Apply a gentle stretch of the arm across the front of the body. Hold the athlete's hand with both hands, bring the athlete's arm straight up to shoulder height, and then cross the athlete's arm over the front of the body to the opposite shoulder.

10. Bring the arm back down to the side of the athlete's body and shake the arm from top to bottom.

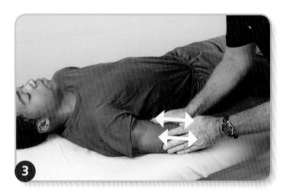

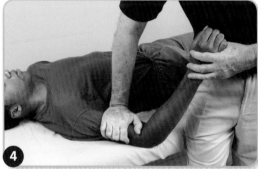

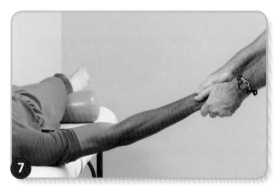

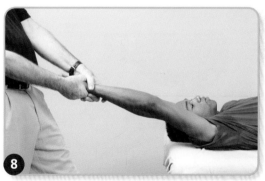

LOWER-BODY PREEVENT ROUTINE

Posterior Lower Body

The routine begins with the athlete lying facedown because the larger, bulkier muscles are on the back side of the lower body. By working up the back side of the lower body in preevent massage and then having the athlete turn over to finish in the face-up position, the trainer can talk to the athlete while finishing the massage. Eye contact is important when communicating with an athlete. The trainer applies steps 1 through 11 to one leg and then repeats the process on the other leg.

1. Apply friction to the calf muscle from the knee to the ankle using brisk back-and-forth motions with both hands for 10 seconds.

2. Apply compression to the calf muscles from the knee to the ankle in three lines, from the outside to the middle and then to the inside of the lower leg. Apply compression strokes three times on each line.

3. Apply lifting, jostling strokes to the calf muscles from the knee to the ankle three times.

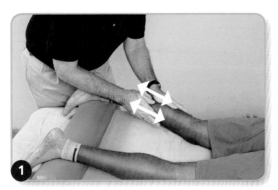

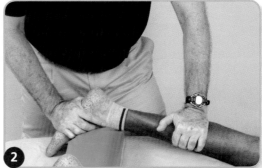

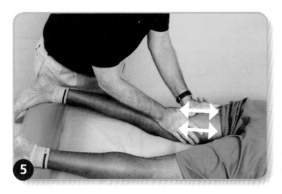

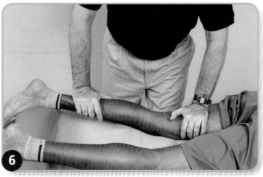

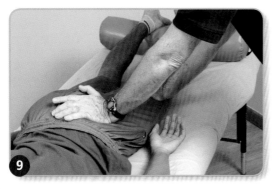

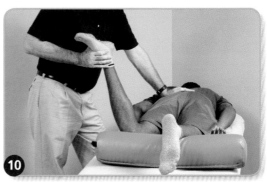

4. Apply shaking to the calf muscles from the knee to the ankle three times.

5. Apply friction to the posterior thigh muscles using brisk back-and-forth motions with both hands from the hip to the knee for 10 seconds.

6. Apply compression to the posterior thigh muscles from the hip to the knee in three lines, from the outside to the middle and then to the inside of the thigh. Apply compression strokes three times on each line.

7. Apply lifting, jostling strokes to the posterior thigh muscles from the hip to the knee three times.

8. Apply shaking to the posterior thigh muscles from the hip to the knee three times.

9. Apply compression to the posterior hip muscles starting at the top of the hip and working around the hip joint three times.

10. Bring the knee to 90 degrees and rock the hip back and forth in internal and external rotation three times.

11. Apply tapotement to the hip and leg three times, starting at the hip and working down the leg.

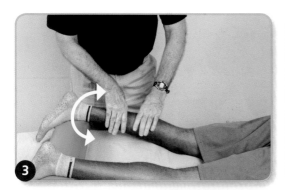

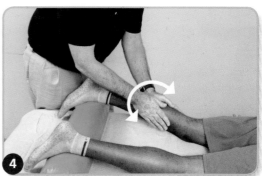

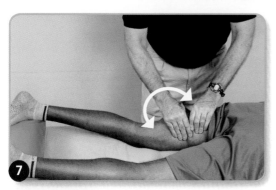

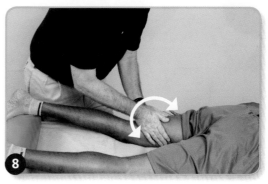

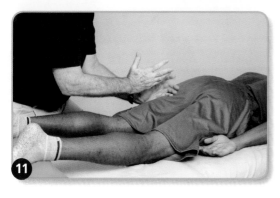

Anterior Lower Body

The trainer has the athlete turn over to the face-up position. The preevent anterior lower body massage can begin on either leg. The trainer applies steps 1 through 11 to one leg and then repeats the process on the other leg.

1. Apply friction to the shin using brisk back-and-forth motions with both hands from the knee to the ankle for 10 seconds.

2. Apply compression to the shin from the knee to the ankle in three lines, from the outside to the middle and then to the inside of the calf. Apply compression strokes three times on each line.

3. Apply lifting, jostling strokes to the shin from the knee to the ankle three times.

4. Apply friction to the thigh using brisk back-and-forth motions with both hands from the hip to the knee for 10 seconds.

5. Apply compression to the thigh from the hip to the knee in three lines, from the outside to the middle and then to the inside of the thigh. Apply compression strokes three times on each line.

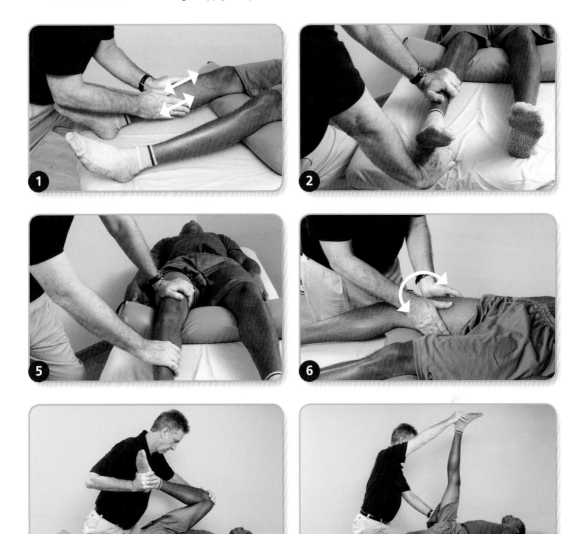

6. Apply lifting, jostling strokes to the thigh from the hip to the knee three times.

7. Apply shaking to the thigh for 10 seconds.

8. Apply stretching to the calf muscles by pushing the ankle toward the head and holding for two seconds. Apply the stretch three times.

9. Apply knee-to-chest range of motion to stretch the posterior hip. Move the knee and hip through their range of motion. Bring the knee from the straight position on the table to the athlete's chest, hold for two seconds, and return to start position. Apply the range of motion three times.

10. Apply a straight leg hamstring stretch. Have the athlete keep the knee locked and lift the straight leg toward the head. Stop when resistance is felt in the forward movement of the leg. Hold for two seconds and then return to starting position. Apply the stretch three times.

11. Apply tapotement to the thigh from the hip to the knee for 10 seconds.

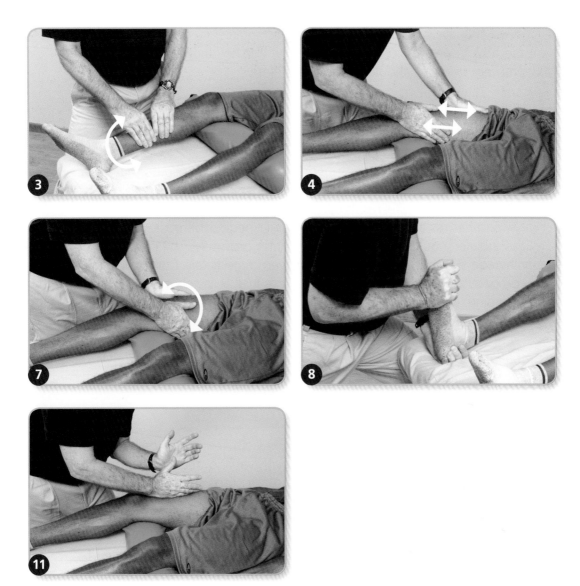

AFTER THE MASSAGE

After performing a preevent sport massage, the trainer may want to assist the athlete up from the massage table. As the athlete sits up, the trainer should look at the athlete's eyes to make sure that the eyes look alert and clear. Sometimes when athletes stand up they can become lightheaded. For this reason the trainer should stand next to the athlete in case he starts to stumble. As the athlete steps away from the table, the trainer should remember to wish him well in the upcoming competition or workout.

The trainer may be the last person to have contact with the athlete before the warm-up and workout or competition. The preevent sport massage should always be pain free, stimulating, and something that the athlete looks forward to experiencing before activity. Preevent sport massage is not just a physical application of sport massage techniques; it is a process of helping the athlete prepare physically, mentally, and emotionally for activity. The preevent massage should inspire the athlete.

POSTEVENT MASSAGE

Postevent sport massage is usually a standard routine. As you will recall from chapter 5, the purpose of a postevent sport massage is to help the athlete recover from a workout or competition. Some time should be allowed after the workout or competition before the postevent massage begins so that the athlete's heart rate, respiratory rate, and body temperature can return to close to her resting rate. Before the trainer begins the postevent massage, the athlete should no longer be perspiring profusely. The postevent sport massage should help the athlete recover immediately from a workout or competition by reducing postexercise soreness, relieving muscle spasm and cramping, enhancing venous return, promoting lymphatic drainage, restoring circulation and flexibility to the muscles, and providing a psychological lift after a competition. The trainer needs to provide the types of treatment that reduce an athlete's postevent exercise soreness but do not treat specific injuries. The techniques for postevent massage are presented in the order of application.

Compressive Effleurage

Effleurage strokes are long gliding strokes applied superficially to deeply. Effleurage strokes are usually applied with varying degrees of pressure. In postevent sport massage the trainer usually starts with lighter effleurage strokes to apply oil and to assess the pain level of the tissues being massaged. On an extremity the trainer wants to surround the arm or leg with the hands and compress the tissue while gliding from distal to proximal. When applied to the back, the trainer starts at the neck and glides down each side of the spine. The mechanical force of effleurage pushes fluid from the extremity into the trunk of the body, allowing fresh blood and lymph to replace the fluid displaced. Compressive effleurage is the major stroke applied to aid recovery in postevent massage because it is thought to push metabolic wastes from the area being massaged.

Petrissage

Petrissage strokes are applied by lifting and squeezing the skin and muscles away from the bone. The intent of petrissage is to milk metabolic waste products, break up adhesions by separating layers of tissue, reduce hypertonicity, reduce muscle soreness, and relieve general fatigue. When petrissage is applied in postevent sport massage, the trainer must not squeeze and lift the muscles too hard because of postexercise soreness. As with compressive effleurage, the trainer starts with lighter pressure and works up to the athlete's tolerance.

Compression

Compression strokes are applied with a rhythmical pumping action to the bellies of muscles. On the extremities, the compression strokes are applied along a line to the outside, straight down, and then to the inside of the extremity. On the back, the compressions are applied up and down the long muscles next to the spine. On the chest, compression strokes are applied to the large pectoral muscles. When applying compression strokes, the trainer should feel the tissue being compressed. The trainer must remember that the tissue can compress only to a certain point before the athlete starts to feel pain. In postevent sport massage the muscles targeted may already be sore, so care must be taken to avoid making the compression strokes painful to the athlete. In addition, various parts of the body are always more tender than others. Muscles on the inside of the thigh, inner arms, and abdomen tend to be softer and more vulnerable to excessive pressure.

Broadening Strokes

Broadening strokes are applied to the bellies of muscles with the hands starting together at the center of the extremity. A downward and outward compressive pressure is applied to the athlete's muscles. The purpose of the broadening strokes is to restore length and broaden the bellies of muscles after exercise. Care must be taken to avoid applying too much downward pressure and to avoid carrying the stroke out too far to the edge of the extremity. The downward pressure can hurt too much, and the outward part of the stroke can pinch the edges of the extremity. Broadening strokes are used primarily on the extremities, working from the upper part of the extremity to the lower part. For example, broadening strokes work well on the anterior thigh and anterior lower leg muscles.

Compressive Effleurage

Starting and finishing with effleurage is soothing to the skin and muscles. The speed and pressure of the technique help inhibit the nerve endings under the area to which compressive effleurage is being applied. Finishing with effleurage also lets the trainer move from one part of the athlete's body to another in a smooth transition. Two important aspects of giving a massage are moving from one part of the body to another smoothly and transitioning from one massage technique to another smoothly. If these transitions are done well, the athlete will not notice the changes and the massage will seem to have a natural flow.

Therapeutic Stretching

Therapeutic stretches are administered at the end of the massage application for any given part of the body. As the body cools down after an event or workout, the athlete may feel a little sore and stiff. The massage often reduces postexercise soreness, but stretching is what restores flexibility and ease of movement. Postevent sport massage stretching should be done gently. Remember that postevent sport massage is done to help the athlete return to a more homeostatic state, or a state of balance. Making the postevent massage stretching experience painful goes against the purpose of the massage.

ADMINISTERING A POSTEVENT MASSAGE

When competing their hardest, athletes often push their bodies beyond the point that is healthy. The trainer never wants an athlete to run right from the finish line to the massage table. The athlete must go through a proper cool-down cycle and be able to respond mentally to postevent massage interview questions. The athlete should be able to answer simple questions like how she is feeling and what part of the body is causing the most difficulty. A postevent sport massage can help the athlete's body begin the recovery process. Before athletes get on the table, the trainer wants them dressed appropriately. For a male athlete, that is usually a pair of shorts. For a female athlete, the appropriate dress is usually a sports bra and shorts.

With the lower-body postevent massage, the trainer is much more likely to encounter problems with cramping in the athlete. Cramping can be handled in several ways. One way is to apply gentle stretches to the muscles that are cramping. If the calf starts cramping, the trainer simply pushes the foot toward the knee and holds to see whether the cramping subsides. Sometimes, the best approach is to have the athlete get up off the massage table and walk around until the cramps subside. If in a worst-case scenario the athlete starts experiencing multiple cramps in various parts of the body, the trainer should call for emergency medical attention.

UPPER-BODY POSTEVENT ROUTINE

Anterior Upper Body

The trainer should start with the athlete lying faceup to permit observation of how the athlete is feeling right after finishing the workout or competition. Observing facial expressions and communicating with the athlete are easier if the athlete is in the face-up position. The trainer should pay attention to the athlete's reaction to the pressure of the massage and the stiffness of the athlete's joints as range of motion is applied. The trainer applies steps 1 through 13 to the forearm, upper arm, and shoulder on one side of the athlete's body and then repeats the process for the forearm, upper arm, and shoulder on the other side.

1. Apply effleurage to the forearm from the wrist to the elbow for 10 seconds.
2. Apply compression strokes to the forearm from the elbow to the wrist three times.
3. Jostling and shaking strokes may be applied to the muscles of the forearm from the elbow to the wrist three times.
4. Massage the palm. The trainer places both thumbs in the middle of the palm and moves the thumbs toward the fingers with a spreading motion. Apply the strokes three times. Then apply range of motion to the wrist. Move the wrist back and forth and side to side three times.

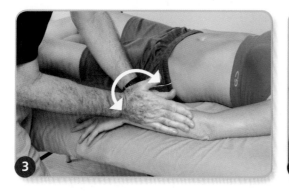

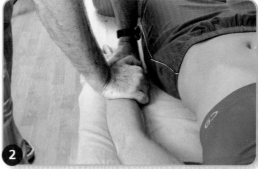

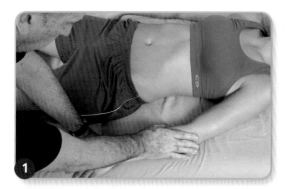

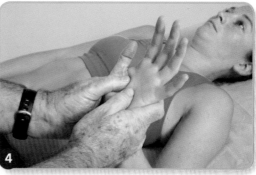

(continued)

Anterior Upper Body   *(continued)*

5. Apply effleurage strokes to the upper arm from the elbow to the shoulder for 10 seconds.

6. Apply compression strokes to the upper arm from the shoulder to the elbow three times.

7. Apply jostling and shaking to the upper arm three times.

8. Apply effleurage to the side of the chest from the sternum out to the shoulder for 10 seconds.

9. Apply compression strokes to the side of the chest from the sternum out to the shoulder three times.

10. Apply range of motion to the arm and shoulder. Grab the athlete's hand and forearm and pull the arm down toward the athlete's feet.

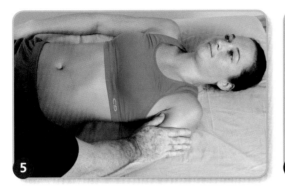

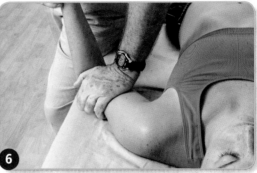

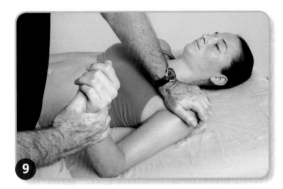

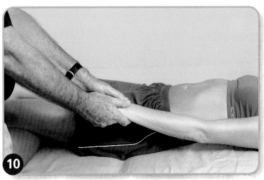

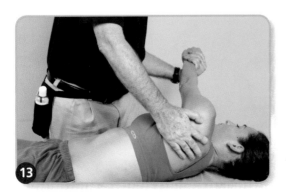

11. Then move the arm to the athlete's shoulder height and pull the arm straight out to the side of the athlete's body.

12. Bring the athlete's arm straight up next to the athlete's head and pull the arm away from the body.

13. Then bring the athlete's arm straight up at the athlete's shoulder height and bring the arm across the athlete's body. Return the athlete's arm to resting position on the massage table.

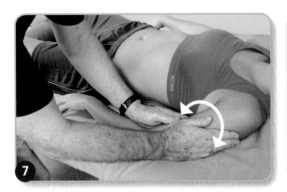

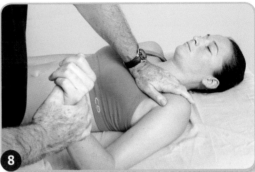

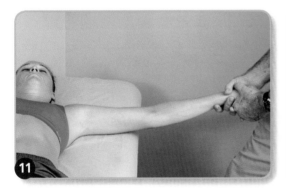

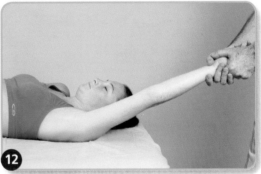

Posterior Upper Body

The trainer is now ready to have the athlete turn over and lie facedown to complete the upper-body postevent massage. When the athlete is in the facedown position, the trainer will not be able to observe the athlete's reaction as easily. The trainer has to pay more attention to how the athlete's body is reacting to massage because the athlete's face will not be visible. The trainer performs steps 1 through 15 to one side of the back and then repeats the process on the other side.

1. Apply effleurage strokes down the back from the shoulder to the hip for 30 seconds. Use both hands on each side of the spine, starting at the shoulders and gliding to the hip. Adjust the pressure to the athlete's comfort level.

2. Apply circular friction from the shoulder to the hip for 30 seconds. Place one hand on top of the other and move in a circular motion.

3. Apply compression next to the spine from the hip to the shoulder. Apply compression strokes three times along this line.

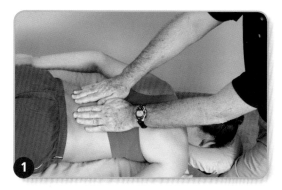

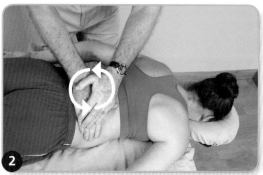

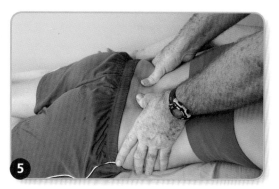

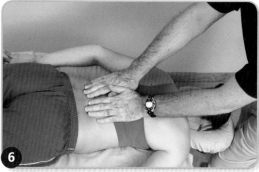

4. Apply compression strokes to the top of both shoulders, starting at the outside of the shoulders and working into the base of the neck. The trainer applies this technique from a standing position at the top of the table.

5. Apply gentle direct pressure on both sides of the spine from the top of the shoulders and down the back. Use the thumbs, holding for 8 to 12 seconds, and adjust the pressure to the athlete's comfort level.

6. Apply compressive effleurage down the back as finishing strokes for 30 seconds. The trainer uses both hands on each side of the spine, starting at the shoulders and gliding to the hip. Pressure is adjusted to the athlete's comfort level.

7. Apply effleurage strokes to the muscles of the anterior side of the forearm from the wrist to the elbow for 10 seconds.

8. Apply compression strokes to the muscles of the anterior forearm from the elbow to the wrist three times.

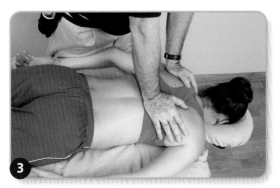

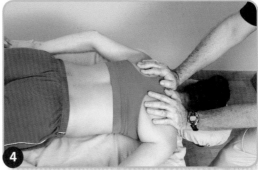

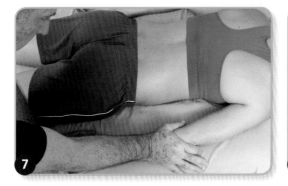

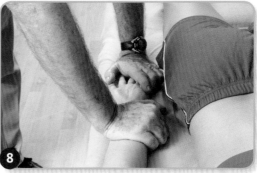

(continued)

Posterior Upper Body   *(continued)*

9. Apply jostling and shaking strokes to the muscles of the anterior forearm three times.

10. Apply compressive effleurage to the upper arm from the elbow to the shoulder for 10 seconds.

11. Apply compression strokes to the upper arm from the shoulder to the elbow three times.

12. Apply jostling and shaking strokes to the upper arm from the elbow to the shoulder for 10 seconds.

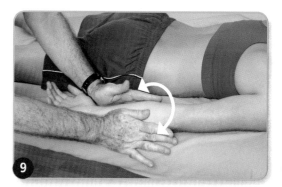

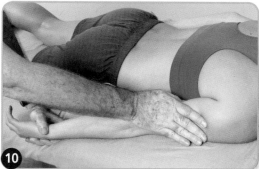

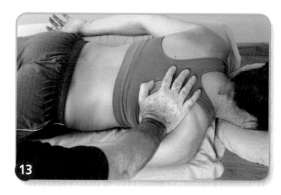

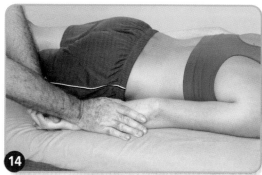

13. Apply compression strokes to the scapula using the palm of one hand in a rhythmical pumping motion.

14. Apply compressive effleurage strokes on the arm from the wrist to the shoulder for 10 seconds.

15. Finish with compressive effleurage strokes down the back.

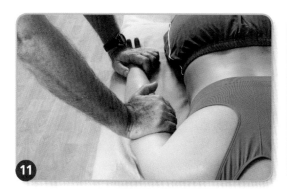

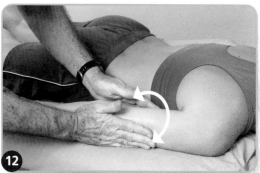

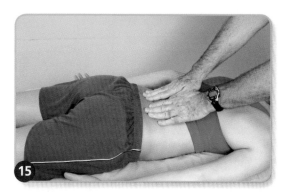

LOWER-BODY POSTEVENT ROUTINE

Anterior Lower Body

The trainer has the athlete turn over to lie faceup and performs steps 1 through 12 on one leg and then repeats the process on the athlete's other leg.

1. Apply compressive effleurage strokes with oil to the anterior lower leg from the ankle to the knee for 10 seconds.
2. Apply petrissage strokes to the anterior lower leg muscles from the knee to ankle. Repeat three times.
3. Apply compression strokes to the anterior lower leg muscles from the knee to the ankle in three lines—outside, top, and inside. Apply the strokes to each line three times.
4. Apply broadening strokes from the knee to the ankle three times.
5. Apply jostling and shaking strokes to the anterior lower leg from the knee to the ankle three times.

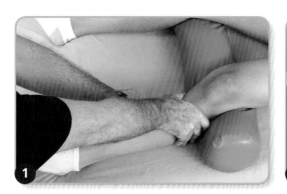

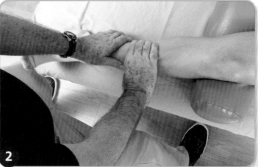

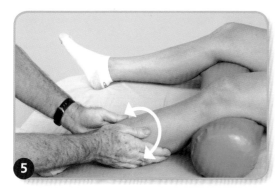

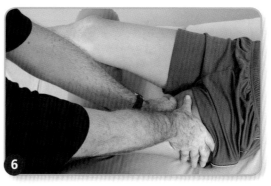

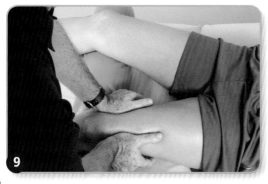

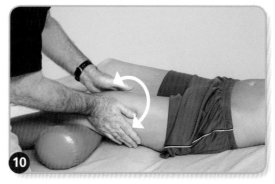

6. Apply effleurage strokes with oil to the anterior thigh from the knee to the hip for 10 seconds.

7. Apply petrissage strokes to the anterior thigh muscles from the hip to the knee in three lines—inside, middle, and outside of thigh. Apply the strokes to each line three times.

8. Apply compression strokes to the anterior thigh muscles from hip to knee along three lines. Repeat each line three times.

9. Apply broadening strokes to the anterior thigh muscles from the hip to the knee.

10. Apply jostling and shaking strokes to the anterior thigh muscles from the hip to the knee three times.

11. Apply knee-to-chest range of motion. After the athlete performs the straight leg raise and has the leg straight in the air, have her or him bend the knee. Then gently push the athlete's knee to the chest. Apply knee-to-chest range of motion three times. Then return the athlete's leg to resting position on the massage table.

12. Apply a straight leg raise. Have the athlete raise the leg straight off the table with the knee locked until the leg stops. Hold for two seconds and return the leg to resting position on the table. Apply the straight leg raise three times.

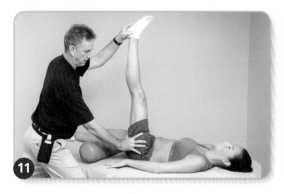

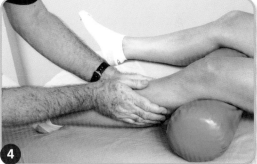

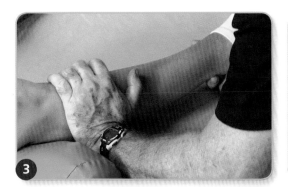

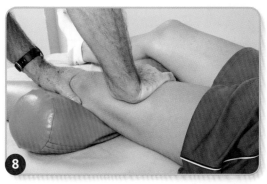

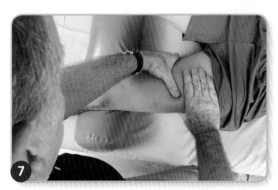

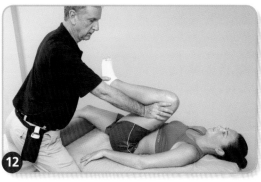

Posterior Lower Body

The trainer has the athlete lie facedown on the table with the feet resting on the bolster. In this position the calf muscles are less likely to cramp. The trainer completes steps 1 through 14 on the leg and hip on one side and then repeats the process on the other side of the athlete's body.

1. Apply compressive effleurage with oil to the calf muscles from the ankle to the knee for 10 seconds.
2. Apply petrissage strokes to the calf muscles from the knee to the ankle three times. Adjust pressure to the athlete's comfort level.
3. Apply compression strokes to the calf muscles from the knee to the ankle in three lines—outside, middle, and inside of the calf. Apply compression strokes three times on each line.

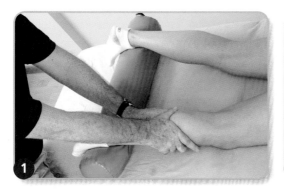
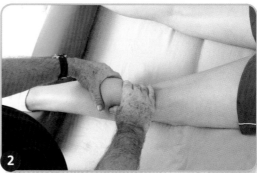
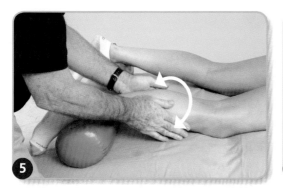
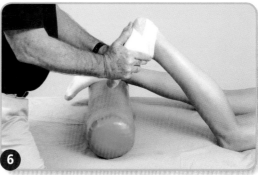

4. Apply broadening strokes to the calf muscles from the knee to the ankle three times.

5. Apply jostling and shaking strokes to the calf muscles from the knee to the ankle three times.

6. Gently stretch the calf muscles by pushing the ball of the foot toward the athlete's head. Hold for two seconds and return the foot to resting position. Apply the stretch three times.

7. Apply compressive effleurage strokes with oil to the posterior thigh muscles from the knee to the hip for 10 seconds.

8. Apply petrissage strokes to the posterior thigh muscles from the hip to the knee along three lines—inside, middle, and outside of the thigh. Adjust the pressure to the athlete's comfort level. Apply petrissage strokes three times along each line.

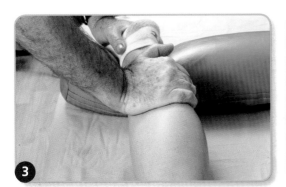

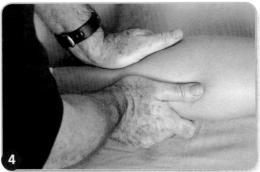

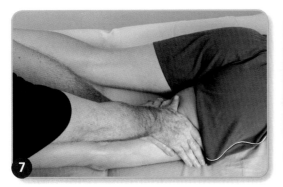

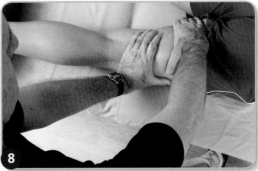

(continued)

Posterior Lower Body *(continued)*

9. Apply compression strokes to the posterior thigh muscles along three lines—inside, middle, and outside. Adjust compression strokes to the comfort level of the athlete and apply them three times.

10. Apply broadening strokes to the posterior thigh muscles from the hip to the knee three times.

11. Apply jostling and shaking strokes to the posterior thigh muscles from the hip to the knee three times.

12. Raise the athlete's leg and move it toward the hip. Gently stretch three times.

13. Apply compression strokes to the posterior thigh muscles with the palm, starting at the top of the posterior hip and compressing around the hip joint.

14. Apply rocking range of motions to the hip. Raise the athlete's leg to 90 degrees with one hand on the athlete's ankle and the other hand on the hip because it compresses hip muscles while rocking. Move the ankle in and out three times. Return the leg to resting position on the massage table.

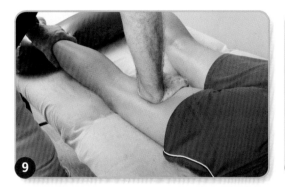

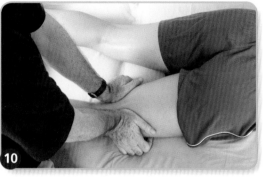

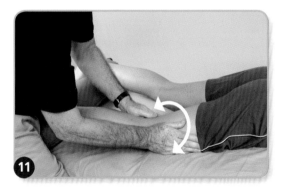

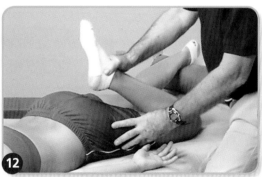

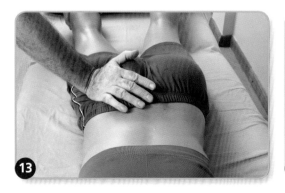

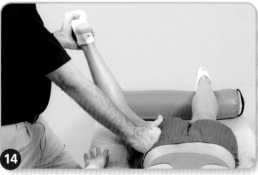

AFTER THE MASSAGE

After performing a postevent sport massage, the trainer may want to assist the athlete up from the massage table. As the athlete sits up, the trainer should look at the athlete's eyes to make sure that her eyes look alert and clear. An athlete who works out or competes to the point of exhaustion may be slightly dehydrated. Sometimes when such an athlete stands up she can become lightheaded. As the athlete begins to use her muscles again in taking the first few steps away from the table, cramping may occur. In very hot or very cold weather, the trainer should make sure that the athlete is dressed appropriately when reentering the environment.

CHAPTER 8

Recovery Massage

The intent of recovery sport massage is to reduce soreness, restore blood flow, increase range of motion, promote lymphatic drainage, and reestablish balance and a sense of well-being. As with postevent massage, applying deep-tissue massage may be inappropriate during a recovery sport massage because it may irritate the athlete's body. A recovery sport massage is usually administered at least one to three days after an event. This interval ensures that the athlete's body has had enough time to achieve a more homeostatic state and has had more opportunity to come back into balance. But even in a period of 24 hours after a long-duration event, an athlete's body is unlikely to recover fully. For that reason, massage during this period is referred to as recovery massage. When athletes complete long-duration workouts or competitions, their bodies may be slightly dehydrated, inflamed, exhausted, injured, and full of endorphins that naturally reduce pain. Thus, athletes cannot sense accurately what effect the massage techniques and therapeutic stretching are having on their bodies. As a result, they cannot give the trainer accurate feedback about the depth and pressure of the massage.

The recovery sport massage can be a full-body massage. Unlike pre- and postevent massage, recovery massage is not done at an event site. The time required to administer the recovery massage is not critical to the intended outcome. Preevent massage usually lasts about 15 minutes, and postevent massage usually lasts no longer than 30 minutes, but recovery massage can take 60 to 90 minutes. The techniques of recovery massage can be done slower and with more depth than they are in event massage. With recovery massage the trainer is trying to find sore, inflamed, tender areas of the athlete's body to help speed the recovery process. The recovery massage techniques are done slower to avoid hurting the athlete, and they are intended to inhibit, soothe, and calm the athlete's nervous system. An athlete might be sore from head to toe in recovery massage or may request only leg or back massage. In recovery massage it should be up to the athlete to decide whether to have a full-body massage or to have parts of the body massaged.

RECOVERY MASSAGE ASSESSMENT

Before providing a recovery massage, the trainer should record the athlete's history and conduct a brief interview. The trainer should make sure that the athlete has had time to rest, rehydrate, and eat before the treatment. Many times, the trainer can tell just by looking whether the athlete is happy, sad, in pain, or excited. Looking at the athlete and really seeing what kind of mood he is in is the first step in assessment for recovery massage. The trainer would not want to be laughing and silly if the athlete is sad, angry, or in pain. The trainer's attitude should adjust to be appropriate to the athlete's needs. Sometimes, the trainer can tell whether a team has won or lost by the demeanor of the athlete in the training room the next day.

A form such as that shown in chapter 1 has a space for the athlete's name, date, and sport. Keeping records of treatments allows the trainer to become more familiar with each athlete and the types of treatments required for each sport. A trainer may see 25 to 30 athletes in one day, and they may come from a variety of team sports for massage. Having an intake form allows the trainer to find out what type of athlete she is working with and where on the body the athlete needs treatment.

When handing an athlete an intake form with a body chart on it, the trainer will often see the athlete move his body in various directions before marking the chart. This process helps the athlete gain body awareness. By knowing which part of the body needs treatment and how sore he is in various parts of the body, the athlete can better communicate that information to the trainer. By listening to the athlete's input, the trainer can adjust the pressure of the massage techniques to match the needs of the athlete's body.

The back of the form should include an area for the trainer to record notes from the assessment, the massage techniques used, and the results of the massage. Nothing can be more frustrating to an athlete than having to explain everything about his body to a new trainer for every treatment. When trainers keep accurate records, others can read what conditions the athlete was treated for previously, what types of massage techniques were used, and how the athlete's body responded to the treatment. Keeping accurate records also allows the trainer to monitor how well the athlete is responding to treatments over a period of weeks.

Three important bits of information to track when recording recovery massage treatments are the athlete's mood (good, bad, or indifferent), the level of pain that the athlete is experiencing (more pain, less pain, or staying the same), and the athlete's joint movement (more range of motion, less range of motion, or staying the same). Recording these three pieces of information allows the trainer to assess the effectiveness of the treatments being administered to the athlete. If the athlete is in a good mood, is in less pain, and is moving the body with ease, then the massage treatments have been effective. The trainer can tell whether an athlete is happy just by looking. The trainer can tell when the athlete is in less pain by watching the athlete move and by noting how the athlete reacts to the pressure of the massage techniques being applied. The trainer can tell when the range of motions is improving by moving the joints during the massage and by watching the athlete's movement after the massage. If the results of the massage treatments are not favorable, then the trainer should sit down with the athlete and discuss how to change the massage treatments.

Looking at how an athlete marks a body chart can help in assessing how the massage should be directed. Questioning the athlete about the way in which he marked the chart can help the trainer give a more effective massage. Athletes often mark the whole back, both legs, and both arms in bold marks across all areas. Bold marks over large areas of the body usually indicate whole-muscle soreness. When treating whole-muscle soreness, nonspecific massage techniques, such as effleurage, petrissage, compression, and broadening strokes, are usually appropriate.

When athletes mark the body chart with small circles or Xs, a specific painful area usually needs treatment. Asking whether the athlete sustained an injury while competing would be advisable. Knowing how long the athlete has had the problem and whether it had been evaluated to determine its cause is important. Diagnosing health-related conditions is not within the scope of practice of a trainer. When an athlete is seeking treatment for a severe condition, the trainer should know whether a doctor has diagnosed the condition.

When no other health care professional is available, the trainer should be cautious when treating an athlete, especially when the athlete is suffering from an acute injury and is in severe pain. Here are some conditions that trainers may often treat in an athletic training room: tender spots, trigger points, overused and stressed muscles, muscle strains, and joint sprains. Knowing exactly what has caused the pain in these conditions is critical to treating them properly.

The scope of this book does not allow teaching in-depth assessment techniques, but conducting a simple direct pressure test can prevent a trainer from performing a massage on an area that should not be treated. The direct pressure test is performed by locating the most sensitive area marked on the chart and applying moderate pressure to the area. When moderate direct pressure is first applied to the sensitive area, the sensation is usually the most intense. With sustained pressure, the intensity should drop off quickly (in about 10 to 12 seconds) because the nervous system and the muscular system respond quickly when stimulated. The nervous system senses the sensations caused by direct pressure, and the muscular system adapts based on how the sensation feels.

If the intensity of the sensations from the moderate direct pressure does not lessen quickly, it may be a sign that the tissue is not capable of functioning properly and that the injury is still in the acute stage. To continue to pressure or stress the painful area would not be advisable. Instead, the trainer should use the RICE treatment, which is the first aid treatment for soft tissue injuries. (Rice stands for rest, ice, compress, and elevate.) If the RICE treatment falls within the trainer's scope of practice, then applying RICE would be appropriate for areas of tenderness in which the sensation does not decrease in intensity with moderate pressure. In most cases with minor aches and pains, the body recovers within 48 to 72 hours. Having the athlete apply ice to an area of tenderness two or three times a day until the tenderness diminishes is appropriate. The trainer can massage around an area of an athlete's body that is too tender to treat directly until that area improves.

RECOVERY MASSAGE TECHNIQUES

When administering recovery sport massage, the techniques should be primarily restorative in nature. Good basic massage techniques with firm pressure should be applied. Recovery sport massage incorporates techniques not used in preevent or postevent massage such as stripping strokes, direct pressure, and cross-fiber friction. Stripping strokes allow trainers to glide through large areas of muscle to determine quickly whether tender areas, trigger points, or tendinitis exists. Direct pressure is applied to the tender areas and held as the sensation goes from sharp to dull. Gentle cross-fiber friction is applied to muscle attachments to reduce soreness of tendons.

Stripping strokes, direct pressure, and cross-fiber friction strokes are added into the recovery massage for their therapeutic effect. They are more invasive massage techniques that the body is better able to handle after a period of rest from a competition or workout. The last thing an athlete would want a trainer to do is poke at her muscles right after having worked out. But after a period of rest, sustained pressure on a muscle often relieves tension. Cross-fiber friction strokes can also be used to reduce muscle soreness and spasms during a recovery massage, but cross-fiber friction should not be used in a preevent or postevent massage because of the possibility of inflaming muscle tissue.

Compressive Effleurage

Compressive effleurage strokes are moderately pressured gliding strokes applied over an extended part of the body. Compressive effleurage strokes can be applied quickly or slowly to stimulate or sedate the nerve endings. Compressive effleurage increases localized circulation by releasing histamines in the body. Histamine release vasodilates the capillary walls. Compressive effleurage enhances venous return by pushing blood using mechanical pressure, and it aids lymphatic movement. Compressive effleurage is one of the most important strokes applied during recovery sport massage.

When performing compressive effleurage, the trainer needs to add oil, lotion, or cream to the body area being massaged. Without a lubricant, the stroke would be irritating because of excess friction between the trainer's hands and the athlete's skin. Learning the exact amount of lubricant to use when massaging each part of the athlete's body takes some practice. The trainer should use enough lubricant to allow the hands to glide over the area being massaged without slipping. The amount of lubricant varies with the type of lubricant used and the type of skin being massaged. If the athlete's skin is dry, a little more lubricant must be used to allow enough glide. Using a little less lubricant to start is best because a little more can always be added during the massage. If the trainer applies too much, he has to wipe off the excess with a towel. The trainer should ask whether the athlete has a preference of lubricants. Some athletes may be allergic to some types of lubricants. The trainer should always ask before applying anything to the athlete's body.

Petrissage

Petrissage strokes, or kneading movements, are applied by picking up, squeezing, and pressing tissue. The application of petrissage can increase blood flow, milk metabolic waste products, break up adhesions by separating layers of tissue, affect the tonus of muscle, reduce muscle soreness, and relieve general fatigue. In recovery sport massage, this technique can help break up adhesions that can form between the layers of tissue as the body cools down during inactivity and sleep.

Compression

Compression strokes target the bellies of muscles and are applied by rhythmical pumping motions with the hand or foot. Compression is accomplished by trapping the muscle bellies between the hand or foot and a hard surface of the body such as bone. The rhythmical pumping action brings blood to the muscle and spreads muscle fibers. Strenuous activity creates postexercise soreness that increases muscle tonus. Increased muscles tonus decreases blood flow and shortens the belly of the muscle. Compression strokes in recovery sport massage are applied to spread muscles fibers, thus increasing blood flow and enhancing the return of the muscle belly to its natural tonus.

Stripping Strokes

Stripping strokes are used to glide through large sections of muscle to locate tender areas. Stripping strokes are performed by applying pressure with the hand or thumb at the insertion (distal) attachment of the muscle and gliding along the muscle to its origin (proximal) attachment. The stripping strokes may be applied as the athlete performs active range of motion.

Here is an example of an application of stripping strokes: Athletes often complain of soreness in their shins in a recovery massage. Stripping strokes are applied by having the athlete dorsiflex the ankle (bring the foot toward the head). The trainer places a thumb on the outside of the lower shinbone (tibia). As the trainer glides the thumb up the outside of the shinbone toward the knee, the athlete points the foot toward the floor. Stripping strokes can be applied three or four times, which can reduce the soreness in the shin. If tender spots are located in the muscle during the application of stripping strokes, the trainer can stop and hold direct pressure over the tender spot until tenderness subsides.

Direct Pressure

After tender areas or trigger points are located, direct pressure is applied to reduce tenderness. Direct pressure is applied by pressing with the thumb, finger, palm, elbow, or foot in one place and holding constant pressure. If comfortable, constant pressure is maintained, and the motor nerve to the muscle responds by adapting to the increased pressure. When direct pressure is removed, the tonus of the muscle decreases, which increases blood flow and range of motion. Direct pressure also increases sensory stimulation in tissue, allowing the athlete to feel a specific area of the body.

Cross-Fiber Friction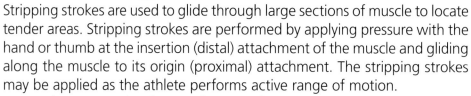

The purpose of cross-fiber friction is to mildly agitate the tissue. This mild agitation can bring blood to the area, break up spasms in muscle, or soften the matrix of forming scar tissue so that the scar is more pliable. Cross-fiber friction, or deep transverse friction, is applied with the fingers or thumb on a muscle, tendon, or ligament on an exact site with firm and consistent pressure. When cross-fiber friction is applied in recovery sport massage, it is usually applied after direct pressure has reduced the level of intensity in the tissue. Cross-fiber friction should not increase the discomfort in the area being treated.

Broadening Strokes

The purpose of a broadening stroke is to flatten out the belly of the muscle widthwise to increase its length. A muscle with more length and width contracts more efficiently. Broadening strokes are applied to the bellies of muscles with the hands together in the center of the muscles. A downward and outward motion is used mostly on the extremities. Broadening strokes may be performed with active range of motion. Broadening strokes in recovery sport massage are usually applied toward the end of the treatment of an area to help the muscle incorporate the more specific massage techniques.

When applying massage techniques to an athlete's body, the trainer starts with the least invasive techniques, moves to the more invasive techniques, and then goes back to the least invasive techniques. Applying massage techniques to the athlete's body this way makes the massage more comforting to the athlete. Broadening strokes with compressive effleurage strokes are great finishing strokes for an extremity of the body.

Jostling and Shaking

Jostling and shaking can stimulate muscle tissue if applied rapidly or ease stress and tension if applied gently. Jostling and shaking strokes are applied by lifting and shaking the skin and muscles of the arms and legs. Jostling and shaking strokes are good finishing strokes for recovery sport massage. Jostling and shaking help prepare the tissue for range of motion and stretching.

Range of Motion

Range of motion techniques are performed by actively or passively moving a joint through its motion. Passive range of motion is often used to stretch and provide sensation to a joint. Active range of motion can be applied while performing other massage techniques to enhance their effects or to provide a stronger stretch. Athletes are often not even aware of soreness in joints and muscles until the trainer moves the joint through various ranges of motion.

Athletes cannot ask the trainer to treat an area of the body if they do not know that it needs treatment. Rocking a joint moves the joint and the muscles attached to it, thus heightening the athlete's awareness of how the joint feels. Range of motion can also help reeducate the muscles after completion of the massage techniques. Before any massage techniques are applied to a muscle, the muscles will have a certain amount of tension. After massage techniques have been applied to a muscle, the tension level within the muscle often changes. When the trainer takes a joint through a range of motion, the nervous system of the athlete's body incorporates the changes in the muscle tension resulting from the massage.

Therapeutic Stretching

Stretching techniques are applied to the body by taking joints through a range of motion. They may be performed with active or passive motions. Active stretches are performed by athletes when they contract their muscles to move a part of the body. Passive stretches are performed when the trainer moves a part of an athlete's body through a range of motion. The purpose of stretching may be to warm up muscles, decrease stiffness, increase range of motion, and rehabilitate injuries. Stretching in recovery sport massage can restore blood flow to muscles, reduce postexercise soreness, and reeducate muscles to return to a natural function.

ADMINISTERING A RECOVERY MASSAGE

A recovery sport massage can last from 30 to 90 minutes, depending on the extent of the massage. Relaxing music may be played during the recovery massage, and the therapist should always be watching for signs of tenderness and pain while administering the massage. Oils or lubricants are used to allow for proper glide when applying the massage techniques. A recovery sport massage may be administered with the athlete wearing little clothing. In this case, proper draping is essential.

Before administering massage, the trainer should review the body chart that the athlete has filled out. Based on the information marked on the chart and the brief interview, the trainer should determine what position the athlete should assume for best treatment. The trainer wants the athlete to be as comfortable as possible from the beginning to the end of the massage. The position in which to start the athlete when applying recovery massage depends on feedback from the athlete. If the athlete is experiencing muscle spasms in a part of the body during the recovery phase, the trainer may want to address that area of the body first so that the athlete is more comfortable during the rest of the massage. Starting a recovery massage with the athlete in the face-up position is usually best because communicating is easier and watching facial expressions is possible.

The recovery massage routines are presented as an upper-body routine and a lower-body routine so that the trainer can choose to do either if not enough time is available to do both. If time permits, recovery massage can be applied to the athlete's whole body. In most cases, the recovery massage starts with the athlete in the face-up position. For a full body massage, the trainer should finish one side of the body before having the athlete turn over because turning back and forth several times is uncomfortable.

UPPER-BODY RECOVERY ROUTINE

Anterior Upper Body

The routine start with the athlete lying faceup (supine) and the palms facing down. A bolster should be placed under the knees of the athlete. The forearms are a good place to introduce recovery massage so that the athlete can feel the massage techniques on the body in a less sensitive area. The recovery massage techniques are applied from the forearm to the hand, to the upper arm, the shoulder, and then the chest. This sequence provides a smooth transition of the massage techniques from one part of the upper body to another. The trainer massages one side of the athlete's body using steps 1 through 23 and then repeats them on the forearm, upper arm, shoulder, and chest on the other side.

1. Apply compressive effleurage to the forearm extensors from the wrist to the elbow 10 times.
2. Apply compression strokes to the forearm extensors from the elbow to the wrist with the palm of the hand three times.
3. Apply stripping strokes to the forearm extensors from the wrist to the elbow. Ask the athlete for feedback about how much pressure to use.
4. Apply direct pressure to the forearm muscles. While applying the stripping strokes, stop anywhere the athlete feels tenderness along the muscle and apply direct pressure. Ask the athlete for feedback about the amount of pressure preferred.

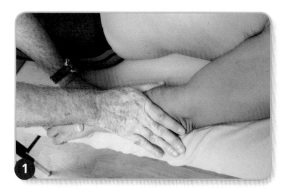

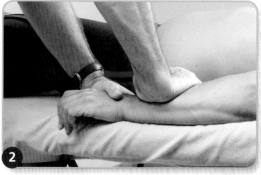

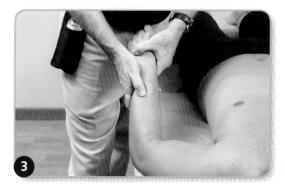

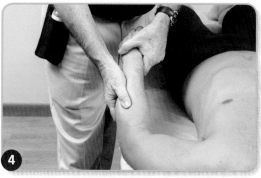

(continued)

Anterior Upper Body   *(continued)*

5. Apply gentle cross-fiber friction to the elbow at the lateral epicondyle (the bony protrusion on the lateral side). Many of the extensor muscles of the wrist originate here. Use the thumb to make small sweeps back and forth over the lateral epicondyle. Adjust the pressure to the athlete's comfort level.

6. Apply broadening strokes to the muscles of the forearm extensors from the elbow to the wrist. Center the palms of the hands in the center of the forearm and spread the palms away from each other toward the outside of the forearm. Adjust the pressure to the athlete's comfort level.

7. Apply jostling and shaking strokes to the muscles of the forearm. To shake the forearm, grasp the athlete's hand and shake the arm from the wrist to the forearm. To jostle the forearm, place the athlete's forearm between the hands and move them back and forth to rock the forearm.

8. Stretch the forearm muscles by flexing the wrist and bringing the palm of the hand toward the forearm. Hold the wrist in the flexed position for two seconds and then straighten. Apply the stretch three times.

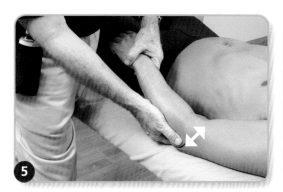

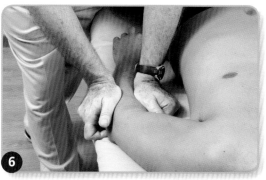

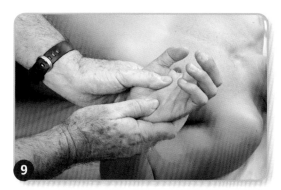

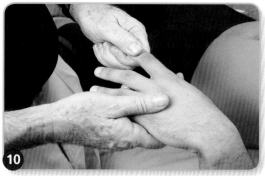

9. Massage the palm with both thumbs. Apply pressure with both thumbs from the wrist in an outward direction to the fingers. Start with the thumbs in the center of the palm and apply multiple stripping strokes from the center of the palm to the outside of the hand.

10. Depending on the sport or position the athlete plays, the fingers and thumb may need treatment as well. With the index finger and thumb, rub the pads between the knuckles of each finger and the thumb. Rub with the finger and thumb in a back-and-forth motion on the pads between the joints.

11. If appropriate, apply range of motion to the fingers and thumb. This is accomplished by gently pushing on the backs of the fingers just above the knuckles. Push the base of the finger toward the palm of the hand. Then with the trainer's thumb on the tip of the athlete's finger move the finger away from the palm of the hand. Gently pull the thumb away from the palm of the hand. All these motions can be completed three times.

12. Apply range of motion to the wrist. Gently move the athlete's wrist back and forth and then side to side. Apply the motions three times.

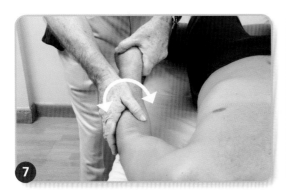
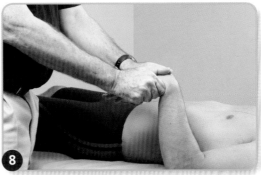
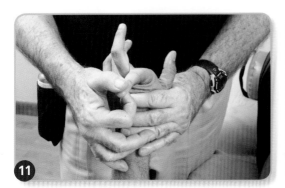
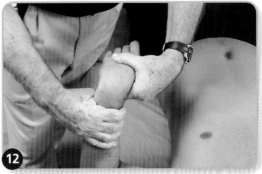

(continued)

Anterior Upper Body *(continued)*

13. Apply effleurage to the upper arm from the elbow to the shoulder. Surround the upper arm with the hand and glide the hand from the elbow to the shoulder with firm pressure.

14. Apply compression strokes to the upper arm from the elbow to the shoulder three times. With the palm apply pressure to the top of the upper arm in a straight line from the shoulder to the elbow. Ask the athlete for feedback about pressure to the upper arm.

15. Apply stripping strokes to the upper arm from just above the elbow to the shoulder. Do not press into the hollow area of the elbow because the artery, veins, and nerves pass through this site. Gentle stripping strokes may be applied to the upper arm from just above the hollow part of the elbow to the shoulder.

16. Apply direct pressure to the upper arm. When applying the gentle stripping strokes to the upper arm, the trainer may stop and apply direct pressure anywhere that a tender spot is encountered. Hold direct pressure on the tender spot for 8 to 12 seconds. The upper arm is often a sensitive area to massage. The pressure on the upper arm should always be comfortable for the athlete.

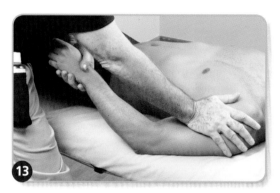

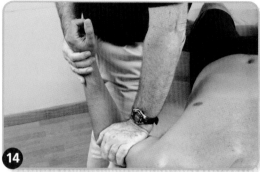

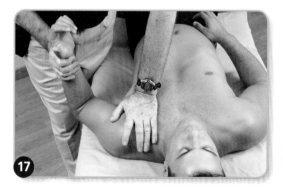

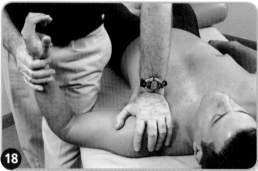

17. Apply compressive effleurage to the chest. Start with the fingers at the breastbone or sternum above the breasts and glide the fingers and then palms of the hands outward toward the shoulders. (When massaging a female athlete, a drape is always maintained over the breasts. Massage the upper chest muscles above the breast and below the collarbone using strokes from the center of the chest to the shoulder.) Apply strokes three times. The chest area can be sensitive on an athlete so ask for feedback about how much pressure to use.

18. Apply compression strokes to the side of the chest with the palm of the hand, working from the breastbone (sternum) in an outward direction toward the shoulder. Apply compression strokes on the chest three times.

19. If needed, apply stripping strokes to the side of the chest. Glide the fingers from the sternum outward toward the shoulder. Work from the lower part of the sternum up to the underside of the collarbone. Where the stripping strokes locate tender points, direct pressure may be held for 8 to 12 seconds. Finish with a few effleurage strokes.

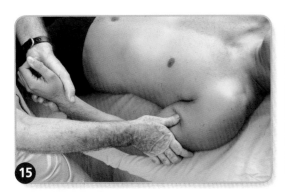

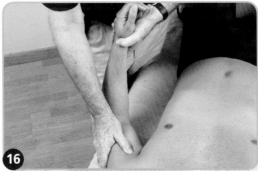

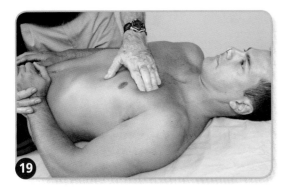

(continued)

Anterior Upper Body *(continued)*

20. Apply range of motion to the arm and shoulder. Range of motion for the shoulder may be applied by grasping the hand and pulling the arm down along the side of the body until it is stretched gently and holding for 10 seconds.

21. Then bring the arm to shoulder level and pull the arm outward away from the athlete's body until it is gently stretched and hold for 10 seconds.

22. Bring arm across body and lift scapula at end of range of motion and hold for 10 seconds.

23. Finally, raise the arm over the athlete's head with the arm next to the ear until it is gently stretched and hold for 10 seconds. Finish range of motion by returning the athlete's arm to the side of the body.

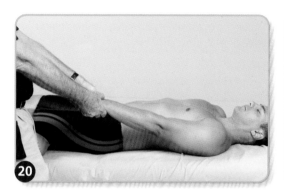

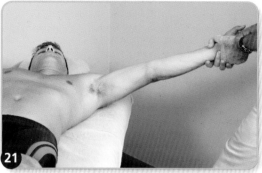

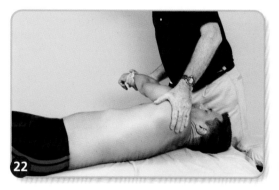

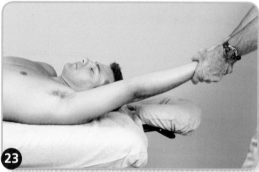

Posterior Upper Body

The trainer now needs to have the athlete move to the facedown position with the arms by the sides and the palms facing up. Before the athlete moves, the trainer takes the bolster out from under knees and inserts the headrest into the end of the massage table. The athlete turns over to lie facedown and places his face in the face cradle at the end of the table. The athlete should be draped appropriately. A bolster placed under the ankles helps relax the legs and prevents the calves from cramping.

1. Apply effleurage strokes down the entire back from the shoulders to the hip. Start with the hands on the athlete's back at the top of the shoulders and perform compressive effleurage strokes down the back to the hips 10 times.

2. Apply circular friction to one side of the back from the shoulder to the hip. Standing on the opposite side of the table from the side being massaged, place one hand on top of the other and make overlapping circular motions down the back from the shoulder to the hip three times.

3. Apply petrissage to the one side of body from the hip to the shoulder by squeezing and lifting the skin and muscle with alternating hands. Apply the strokes three times.

4. Apply compression on the side of the back next to the spine from the hip to the shoulder. Standing on the opposite side of the table, use the palm of the hand on the opposite side of the spine. Start with the palm just above the hip and right next to the spinous process of the back. Apply multiple compression strokes from the hip up the back along the spine to the shoulders. Apply the strokes three times.

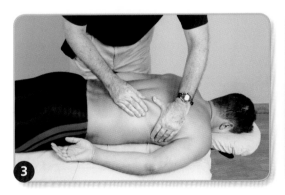
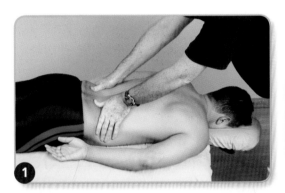
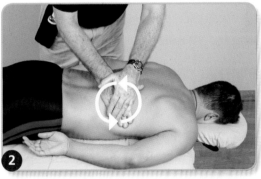
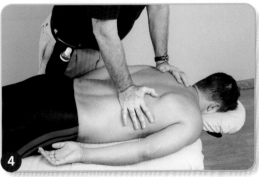

(continued)

Posterior Upper Body *(continued)*

5. From the top of the table, apply compression strokes to the top of both shoulders. Standing at the top of the table with the hands on the outside of the athlete's shoulders, begin pushing the shoulders with the palms straight down toward the feet. Apply compression strokes, moving the hands from the outside of the shoulders along the top to the base of the neck. Apply a compression stroke and then move the hands inward toward the neck. Apply the strokes three times.

6. Apply gentle, direct thumb pressure along the top of the shoulders to the neck. Apply pressure three times, holding for two seconds each time.

7. Apply direct pressure on each side of the spine from the shoulders to the top of the sacrum. Apply direct pressure along the spine three times, adjusting the pressure to the athlete's comfort level and holding the pressure for two seconds each time.

8. To finish, apply compressive effleurage down the back along the spine 10 times. Adjust the pressure to the comfort level of the athlete.

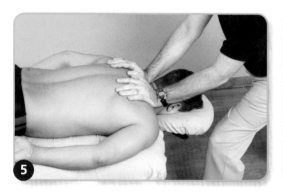

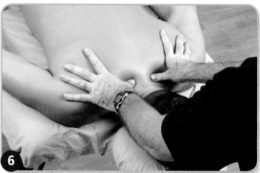

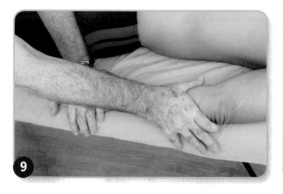

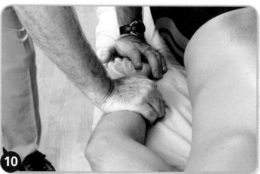

The trainer repeats steps 1 through 8, focusing on the other side of the back. The trainer then completes the next steps (9 through 20) on one arm and then the other.

9. Apply effleurage strokes to the muscles of the side of the forearm starting at the wrist and gliding to the elbow. Apply the strokes 10 times.

10. Apply compression strokes with the palm to the muscles of the side of the forearm from the elbow to the wrist. Remember that compression strokes are rhythmical pumping actions directed at the bellies of the muscles. Apply the strokes three times.

11. Apply stripping strokes to the muscles of the forearm from the wrist to the elbow. Ask the athlete about whether to apply more or less pressure. Stripping strokes are also used for locating tender points along the muscles of the forearm.

12. Apply direct pressure to the forearm muscles. When applying the stripping strokes, the trainer can apply direct pressure anywhere the athlete feels tenderness. Again, the trainer should ask the athlete for feedback about how much pressure to apply. Hold direct pressure for two to four seconds. The tenderness should go from sharp to dull as the tender spots are held.

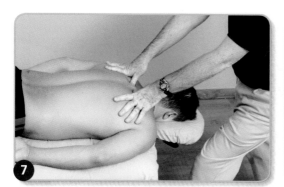

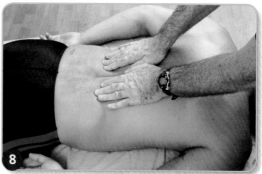

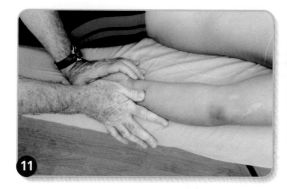

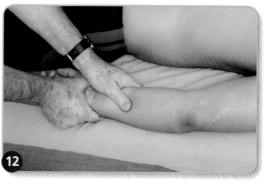

(continued)

Posterior Upper Body   *(continued)*

13. Apply broadening strokes to the muscles of the forearm from the elbow to the wrist. Broadening strokes are applied by centering the palms of the hands in the center of the forearm and spreading the palms away from each other toward the outsides of the forearm. Pressure should be adjusted to athlete's comfort level.

14. Apply jostling and shaking strokes to the muscles of the side of the forearm. Jostling strokes are applied by placing the forearm between the hands and moving the hands back and forth to rock the forearm. Shaking can be applied to the forearm by grasping the athlete's hand with both hands and shaking the arm from the wrist to the forearm.

15. Apply compressive effleurage to the upper arm from the elbow to the shoulder. Surround the upper arm with the hands and glide the hands from the elbow to the shoulder with firm pressure. Apply the strokes 10 times.

16. Apply compression strokes to the upper arm from the shoulder to the elbow. With the palm of the hand apply pressure to the top of the upper arm in a straight line from the shoulder to the elbow. Ask the athlete for feedback on pressure to the upper arm. Apply the strokes three times.

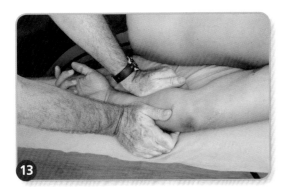
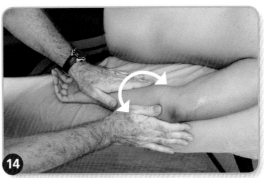

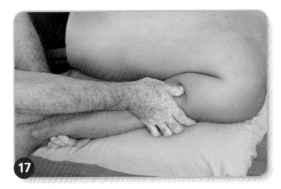
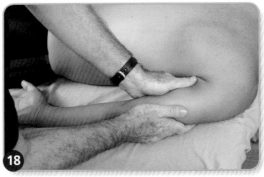

17. Using the thumbs, apply gentle stripping strokes to the upper arm muscles from the elbow to the shoulder three times.

18. Apply broadening strokes to the upper arm. Broadening strokes are applied by placing both palms in the center of the upper arm and spreading the palms away from each other toward the outside of the upper arm. Repeat three times.

19. Apply jostling and shaking strokes to the upper arm from the elbow to the shoulder. Jostling strokes are applied by placing the upper arm between the hands and moving the hands back and forth to rock the upper arm. Shaking can be applied to the upper arm by grasping the athlete's hand with both hands and shaking the arm from the wrist to the upper arm.

20. Finish massaging the arm with compressive effleurage strokes from the wrist to the shoulder. Adjust the pressure to the athlete's comfort level. Apply the strokes 10 times.

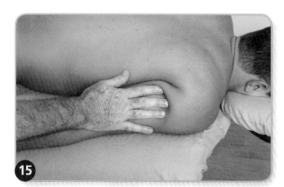

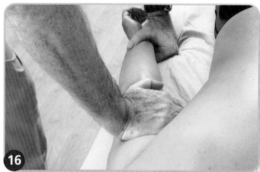

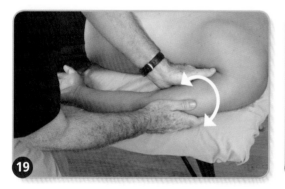

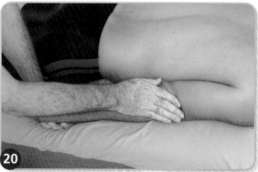

LOWER-BODY RECOVERY ROUTINE

Anterior Lower Body

The athlete lies faceup on the table with the palms down. The back of the athlete's head rests comfortably on the massage table. A bolster is placed under the athlete's knees. The trainer is now ready to perform the recovery massage to the anterior portion of the lower body. The trainer performs steps 1 through 17 to the lower leg, thigh, and hip on one side and then repeats the steps on the athlete's other side.

1. Using both hands, apply compressive effleurage to the lower leg from the ankle to the knee 10 times. Adjust the pressure to athlete's comfort level.

2. Apply petrissage to the inside of the lower leg muscles from the knee to the ankle three times.

3. Apply compression strokes to the outside, top, and inside of the lower leg three times. Adjust the pressure of the compression strokes to the comfort level of the athlete.

4. Apply stripping strokes to the outside, top, and inside of the lower leg. Glide the thumbs from the ankle to the knee. Apply stripping strokes in each of the three lines three times.

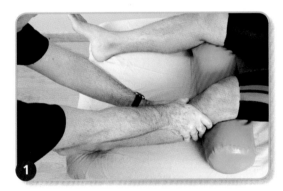

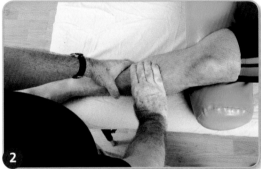

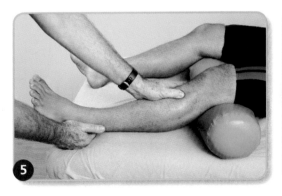

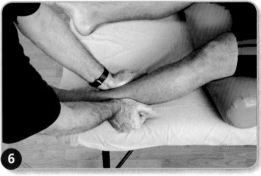

5. Apply direct pressure to the muscles from the ankle to the knee. When performing the stripping strokes, stop at any tender areas and apply direct pressure. Hold direct pressure over tender areas for two to four seconds. Tenderness should go from sharp to dull as the spots are held. Check with the athlete for comfort level with direct pressure.

6. Apply broadening strokes to the lower leg from the knee to the ankle. With the palms together in the center of the upper lower leg, apply pressure downward and outward. Apply strokes three times and adjust the pressure to the athlete's comfort level.

7. Apply jostling and shaking strokes to the lower leg. Jostling strokes are applied by placing the lower leg between the hands and moving the hands back and forth to rock the lower leg. Shaking can be applied by grasping the athlete's lower leg with both hands and shaking it from the knee to the ankle.

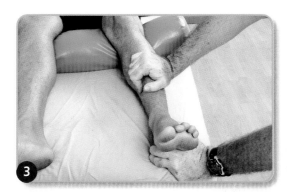

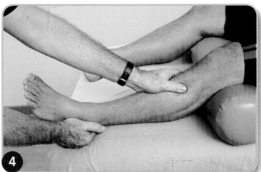

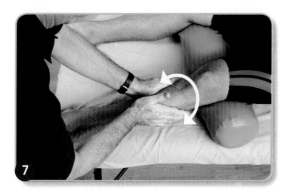

(continued)

Anterior Lower Body   *(continued)*

8. Apply a gentle stretch to the lower leg. Place the hand on top of the foot and gently press the ankle toward the table until it stops. Hold for two seconds and then release the pressure. Apply the stretch three times

9. Apply compressive effleurage to the thigh muscles from the knee to the hip 10 times.

10. Apply petrissage strokes to the thigh muscles. Apply compression strokes to the thigh muscles from the hip to the knee on the outside of the thigh, on the top of the thigh, and on the inside of the thigh. Apply compression strokes in three lines three times. Adjust the pressure of the strokes to the athlete's comfort level.

11. Apply compression strokes to the outside, top, and inside of thigh muscles three times.

12. Apply stripping strokes to the thigh muscles by gliding the thumbs from the knee to the hip on the outside of the thigh, along the top of the thigh, and on the inside of the thigh. Apply stripping strokes in three lines three times.

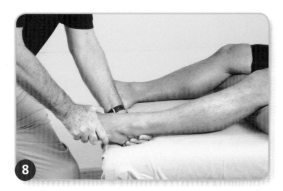

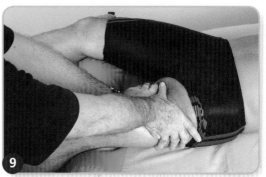

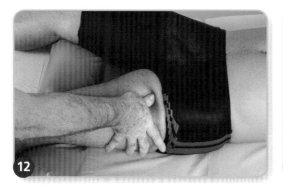

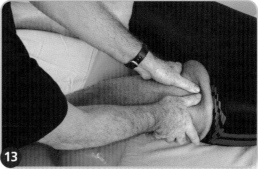

13. Apply direct pressure to the thigh muscles from the knee to the hip. When performing the stripping strokes, stop at any tender areas and apply direct pressure. Hold direct pressure over tender areas for eight seconds. Tenderness should go from sharp to dull as the tender spots are held. Check with the athlete for comfort level with direct pressure.

14. Apply broadening strokes to the thigh muscles from the hip to the knee. With the palms together in the center of the upper thigh muscles, apply pressure downward and outward. Apply strokes three times and adjust the pressure to the athlete's comfort level.

15. Apply jostling and shaking strokes to the thigh muscles. Jostling strokes are applied by placing the thigh between the hands and moving the hands back and forth to rock the thigh. Shaking can be applied by grasping the thigh and shaking from the top of the thigh down to the knee.

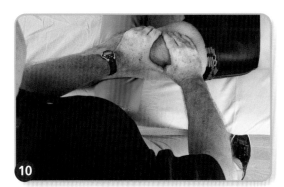

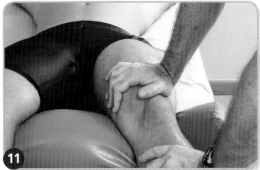

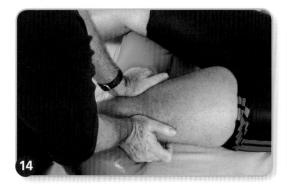

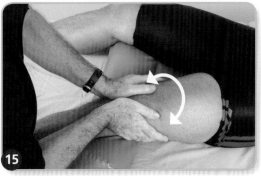

(continued)

Anterior Lower Body   *(continued)*

16. Apply knee-to-chest range of motion to the leg. Have the athlete bring the knee to the chest with the knee bent. Gently push the knee toward the chest and hold for two seconds. Bring the leg back to the resting position to the table. Apply the stretch three times.

17. Apply a straight leg raise to the leg. Have the athlete lift the leg with the knee locked straight up and bring the leg toward the athlete's head. Assist the athlete in a gentle stretch. Hold for two seconds and return the leg to the resting position back on the table. Apply the stretch three times.

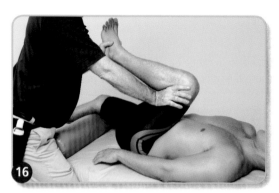

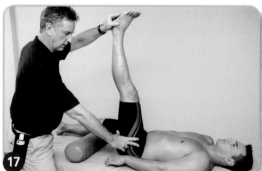

Posterior Lower Body

After removing the bolster from under the knees, the trainer should have the athlete turn over to the facedown position and move up on the table until the athlete's face can rest comfortably in the face cradle at the top of the table. The trainer places a bolster under the athlete's ankles. The trainer performs steps 1 through 21 to the lower leg, thigh, and hip on one side and then repeats the steps on the athlete's other side.

1. Apply compressive effleurage to the calf muscles from the ankle to the knee 10 times.
2. Apply petrissage strokes to the calf muscles from the knee to the ankle three times.
3. Apply compression strokes to the calf muscles from the knee to the ankle three times. Adjust the pressure to the comfort level of the athlete.
4. Apply stripping strokes to the calf muscles from the ankle to the knee by gliding the thumbs. Do not apply pressure into the hollow space behind the knee because the arteries, veins, and nerves pass through that space, although rubbing the space is OK. Apply the strokes three times.

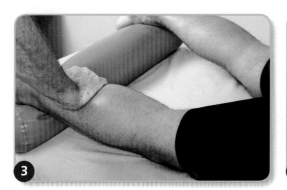

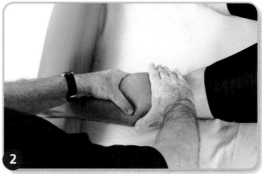

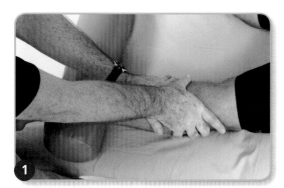

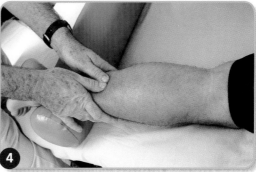

(continued)

Posterior Lower Body   *(continued)*

5. Apply direct pressure to the calf muscles from the ankle to the knee. Stop at any tender areas and apply direct pressure for eight seconds. Tenderness should go from sharp to dull as the tender spots are being held. Check with the athlete for comfort level.

6. Apply broadening strokes to the calf muscles from the knee to the ankle three times. With the palms of the hands together in the center of the upper calf, apply pressure downward and outward. Adjust the pressure to the athlete's comfort level.

7. To finish the massage strokes, apply compressive effleurage strokes to the calf muscles from the ankle to the knee 10 times.

8. Apply jostling and shaking strokes to the calf muscles from the knee to the ankle. Jostling strokes are applied by placing the calf between the hands and moving the hands back and forth to rock the calf muscles. Shaking can be applied to the calf muscles by grasping the athlete's calf with both hands and shaking the calf from the knee to the ankle.

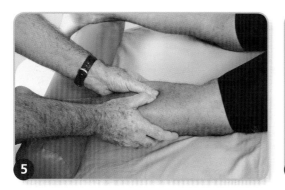

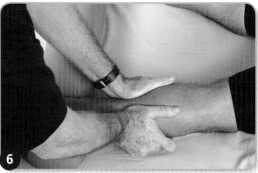

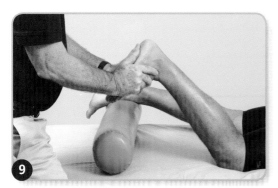

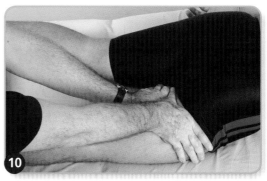

9. Apply a gentle stretch to the calf muscles. Lift the lower leg about 45 degrees off the table. Place the hands on the athlete's foot and ankle and press the ankle toward the athlete's head until the stretch is felt. Hold in stretched position for two seconds and then let off the pressure. Apply the stretch three times.

10. Apply compressive effleurage strokes to the thigh muscles (hamstrings) from the knee to the hip 10 times.

11. Apply petrissage strokes to the thigh muscles from the hip to the knee three times.

12. Apply compression strokes to the thigh muscles from the hip to the knee three times. Adjust the pressure to the athlete's comfort level.

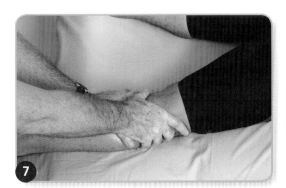

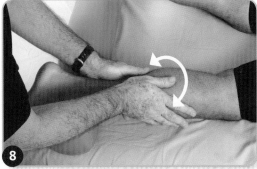

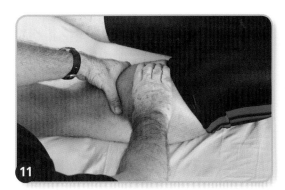

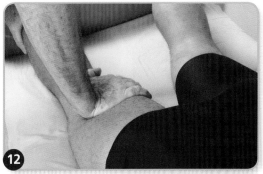

(continued)

Posterior Lower Body *(continued)*

13. Apply stripping strokes to the thigh muscles from the knee to the hip. Glide the thumbs from the upper part of the hollow space behind the knee to the hip. Do not apply pressure into the hollow space behind the knee because the arteries, veins, and nerves pass through that space, although rubbing the space is OK. Apply the strokes three times.

14. Apply direct pressure to the thigh muscles from the knee to the hip, stopping at any tender areas to apply direct pressure for eight seconds. Tenderness should go from sharp to dull as the tender spots are held. Check with the athlete for comfort level.

15. Apply broadening strokes to the thigh muscles. With the palms together in the center of the upper thigh muscles, apply pressure downward and outward on the thigh from the hip to the knee three times. Adjust the pressure to the athlete's comfort level.

16. Apply jostling and shaking strokes to the thigh muscles. Jostling strokes are applied by placing the thigh between the hands and moving the hands back and forth to rock the thigh. Shaking can be applied by grasping the athlete's thigh with both hands and shaking the thigh from the hip to the knee.

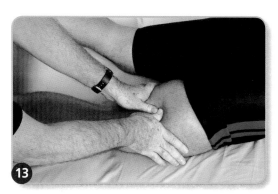

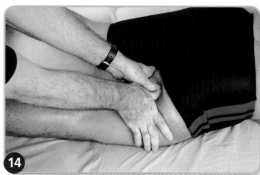

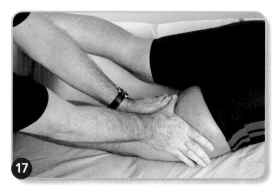

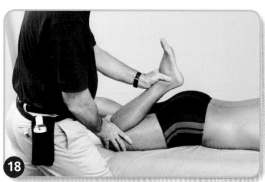

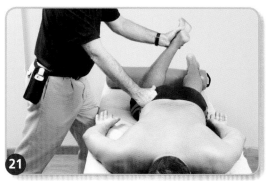

17. Finish the massage strokes on the thigh by applying compressive effleurage from the ankle to the hip 10 times.

18. Apply range of motion to the knee. Lift the ankle to 90 degrees and bring the ankle toward the hip until a stretch is felt. Hold for two seconds and release the pressure. Apply range of motion three times.

19. Apply compression to the hip muscles. With the palm of the hand, press in to the hip around the hip joint three times.

20. Apply compression to the hip muscles with the flats of the hands. With the fingers folded over to the palm of the hand, press with the backs of the fingers around the hip joint. Apply the strokes three times.

21. Apply rocking range of motions to the hip. Put one hand around the ankle, while the other hand compresses the hip muscles, and bring the lower leg straight to 90 degrees. With the lower leg in the 90-degree position, rock the thigh in and out, rotating the hip socket gently until the hip stretches in both directions. Drop the lower leg back on the table to resting position.

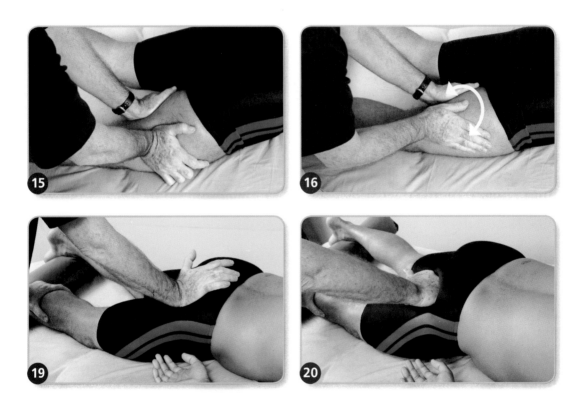

AFTER THE MASSAGE

After performing a recovery sport massage, the trainer may want to help the athlete up from the massage table. As the athlete sits up, the trainer should look at the athlete's eyes to make sure that they look alert and clear. The athlete may need a few minutes to become alert, so the trainer should not rush him off the table. Conducting a brief interview with the athlete after the massage is helpful in determining whether the intent of the massage was accomplished. The trainer should ask the athlete how he feels after the massage and make sure that all the major issues were addressed.

The trainer should watch the athlete walk away from the table to make sure that he is not feeling lightheaded and has good balance. If the athlete feels lightheaded, the trainer should have him sit back down for a few minutes until the athlete feels better. A suggestion to ice any areas of residual soreness and a reminder to drink fluids for proper rehydration may be appropriate. Most athletes are familiar with the application of ice to the body. The ice treatment lasts 20 minutes and is used to reduce inflammation and soreness after exercise. Increased water intake may help the kidneys flush metabolic waste products from the body.

CHAPTER 9

Sport-Specific Treatments

The purpose of this chapter is to help the trainer understand how to apply sport massage to athletes who are participating in specific sports. The trainer will learn how participation in specific sports can affect specific parts of an athlete's body, what kind of muscle and joint problems can develop from playing various sports, what types of massage techniques are effective for treating specific problem areas, and which stretches or range of motion movements can be applied after treatment. The purpose of this chapter is not to diagnose athletic injuries, but to bring attention to common conditions that occur in the athlete's body that a trainer must learn to assess and treat.

Most massage treatments for specific areas of the body should last about 15 minutes. The massage techniques used in a treatment should always start with the nonspecific massage techniques to warm up the superficial tissue over the area being treated. Next, the more specific massage techniques directed at the targeted tissue are applied to achieve the therapeutic result intended. Finally, the more superficial massage techniques are used to soothe the area at the end of the treatment. A light touch to an athlete's tissue that causes the athlete to wince is usually a sign that the tissue is in an acutely inflamed state. Massage is contraindicated on the direct site of injury during the acute stage. Ice applications or topical analgesics may be applied until the acute stage of injury subsides. This process usually takes 48 to 72 hours.

COMMON PROBLEM AREAS IN SPORT

Before we get into sport massage techniques for specific sports, we note that trainers should be able to recognize general areas on athletes' bodies that can become strained and overused from physical activity. Movements common to most sports like running, jumping, kicking, throwing, and swinging an object like a bat or golf club cause stress to specific parts of the athlete's body. Trainers should know the specific places on an athlete's body stressed by those common movements. Because this book cannot cover specific sport massage applications for every sport, let's look at areas of the body that typically require attention no matter what sport the athlete participates in.

Our approach to this section is to identify the area of the body that we are looking at, the stresses that affect that area, the massage techniques that can be administered to the area, and stretching and ranges of motion that can be used to complete the treatment for that area of the body. We will start with the strains that commonly occur in the foot and work our way up through the athlete's body.

Feet

The feet are usually a good place to start because in most sport applications they are the first part of an athlete's body to strike the ground. When the feet strike the ground, they should provide a stable platform for all the joints above. If an athlete cannot plant the foot and put his or her weight over it with confidence, moving effectively is extremely difficult. The bottoms of the feet often become sore and tender. A condition known as plantar fasciitis can occur, making every step that an athlete takes painful. Plantar fasciitis is an irritation of the dense fibrous band of connective tissue on the bottom of the foot that originates at the heel and extends to the toes. The condition can be caused by an increase in running mileage, an increase in training intensity, running up hills, or a breakdown in running shoes.

The foot and ankle go through three stages of movement during running. The first stage, called the heel strike, occurs when the lateral part of the heel makes contact with the ground. The second stage is midstance. The weight of the runner's body moves from the lateral heel to the bottom of the foot. The third stage is toe-off. The weight of the athlete's body moves to the ball of the foot as she or he propels the body forward. From heel strike to toe-off, the plantar fascia tightens on the bottom of the athlete's foot. Any awkward motions of the ankle or foot that stress the bottom of the foot can cause the plantar fascia to become inflamed.

Massage is difficult when the plantar fascia is extremely inflamed. Soaking the foot in cold water for 20 minutes three times a day and reducing running activity can help relieve inflammation of the plantar fascia. After treatment to reduce the inflammation has been successful, massaging the bottom of the foot may begin. Massage strokes used for treating plantar fasciitis are compressive effleurage, flats of hands, stripping strokes, direct pressure, cross-fiber friction, and compressive effleurage to finish.

With the athlete lying facedown with a bolster under the ankles, the trainer begins massage of the bottom of the foot with firm effleurage strokes from the toes to the heel using a small amount of Prossage Heat, just enough to allow the hands to glide over the skin of the bottom of the foot without slipping. The trainer applies 10 effleurage strokes to the bottom of the foot and then applies five flats of hands on the bottom of the foot from the heel to the ball of the foot. The trainer then applies stripping strokes from the ball of the foot to the heel with the thumb, starting on the inside of the foot and moving to the outside of the foot and stripping through the entire bottom of the foot three times. Stripping strokes start with light pressure and then the pressure is increased to the athlete's tolerance. When performing the stripping strokes, the trainer may stop at any tender areas and hold direct pressure until the tenderness subsides. Direct pressure is held for 8 to 12 seconds. Next comes cross-fiber friction to the distal part of the heel on the bottom of the foot. The cross-fiber friction technique applied to the heel should always reduce discomfort to the tissue, not increase it. Cross-fiber friction is applied for 30 seconds, and the massage ends with compressive effleurage strokes on the bottom of the foot.

To finish the treatment, stretches should be applied to the calf and the bottom of the foot. To stretch the calf, the athlete dorsiflexes the ankle (brings the toes toward the nose), holds in the stretched position for two seconds, and then releases. The stretch is performed eight times. Next, the athlete pulls the toes into extension (brings the toes toward the top of the foot), holds in the stretched position for two seconds, and then releases. The stretch is performed eight times. If residual soreness is still present, topical analgesic should be applied to the bottom of the foot three times a day. This treatment may be applied every other day until the condition improves.

Lower Legs

In the lower leg, muscles close to the shin often become tender. A condition known as shin splints can cause pain along the anterior shin (anterior shin splints) or pain along the posterior shin (posterior shin splints). Shin splints are simply pain and discomfort in the lower leg from repetitive activity. The overuse of the tibialis anterior or the tibialis posterior muscles stresses the tendinous attachments and causes the muscles to spasm. Shin splints can occur for many reasons, but the most common one is overuse of the muscles of the lower leg from increasing running mileage or adding intensity to workouts. Attempting to massage these muscles when they are acutely inflamed is not recommended. Soaking the lower leg in cold water for 20 minutes three times a day and reducing stress on the lower leg by decreasing mileage until the condition improves is recommended. After treatment to reduce the inflammation has been successful, massage of the lower leg may begin.

Massage strokes used for treating shin splints are compressive effleurage, stripping strokes, direct pressure, cross-fiber friction, broadening strokes, and compressive effleurage to finish. To begin, the athlete lies faceup on the massage table with a bolster under the knees. The massage starts with 10 compressive effleurage strokes to the lower leg from the ankle to the knee using a small amount of Prossage Heat. Next, stripping strokes are applied from the ankle to the knee along both anterior and posterior sides of the shin (tibia). While performing the stripping strokes, the trainer may stop at any tender areas and hold direct pressure until the tenderness subsides. Direct pressure is held for 8 to 12 seconds.

As the tenderness decreases, friction should be applied along the shin with the fingers on one side of the tibia and the thumb on the other. The friction pressure should be adjusted to the athlete's comfort level. The application of the friction technique may reduce spasming along the muscle attachments. As the condition improves, the trainer can have the athlete move the ankle up and down while the friction technique is being applied to the shin. The trainer then moves from the friction technique to broadening strokes, starting at the top of the shin and working down to the ankle. The massage techniques to the lower leg end with compressive effleurage strokes.

To finish the treatment, stretches should be applied to the lower leg. As the athlete dorsiflexes the ankle (brings the toes to the nose), the trainer pushes on the ball of the foot and holds for two seconds. The athlete then plantarflexes the ankle (points the foot down toward the table), and the trainer presses on the top of the foot and holds for two seconds. The athlete alternates stretches, holding in each direction for two seconds and then releasing. Lower leg stretches are performed eight times. If residual soreness is still present, a topical analgesic should be applied three times a day on alternating days until the condition improves.

Anterior Thighs

The muscle group on the front and lateral aspect of the thigh is called the quadriceps group. The quadriceps muscles are powerful muscles that extend the knee in running, jumping, and kicking motions. Often, they become sore because of overuse, after intense workouts, or after weightlifting exercises like squats. Of the four quadriceps muscles, the vastus lateralis, the quadriceps muscle along the outside of the thigh, is most often sore in athletes.

Massage strokes used for treating the quadriceps muscles are compressive effleurage, petrissage, compression strokes, stripping strokes, direct pressure, broadening strokes, and compressive effleurage to finish. The athlete lies in the face-up position with a bolster under the knees. The massage begins with compressive effleurage using a small amount of Prossage Heat. Strokes are applied from the knee to the top of the thigh 10 times. Next, petrissage is applied to the quadriceps muscles on the inside, top, and outside of the thigh, using three passes over each area. The trainer then applies compression strokes in the same areas, inside, top, and outside of the thigh, three times. Stripping strokes are then applied to the same three areas, using three passes in each area. While performing the stripping strokes, the trainer may stop at any tender areas and hold direct pressure for 8 to 12 seconds until the tenderness subsides. The vastus lateralis muscle is likely to have numerous trigger points along the entire muscle from the hip to the knee. When performing stripping strokes and direct pressure to the vastus lateralis, the trainer should be sure that the amount of pressure is comfortable to the athlete. After stripping strokes and direct pressure, the trainer applies broadening strokes from the hip down the thigh to the knee three times. The massage ends with compressive effleurage strokes from the knee to the hip 10 times.

To finish the treatment, stretches should be applied to the quadriceps muscles. The athlete turns to the side-lying position on the massage table and flexes the bottom knee to the chest. The athlete holds the ankle of the top leg and brings the knee of the top leg to the chest. The athlete extends the top knee until it is in a straight line with the rest of the body, holds the stretch for two seconds, and then brings the knee back to the chest. The stretch is performed eight times. If residual soreness is still present in the quadriceps muscles, a topical analgesic can be applied to the thigh three times a day on alternating days until the condition improves.

Hips

The deep posterior hip muscles are referred to as the six deep lateral rotators. These muscles are often tight on athletes. Tight lateral rotators are often noticeable because they cause the feet to rotate outward when an athlete is walking or running. Activities like running, jumping, and kicking can aggravate the six deep lateral rotators. The piriformis, one of these lateral rotators, is located between the sacrum and the hip and is a primary source of posterior hip discomfort. The piriformis can create pain in the hip in three different ways. First, the muscle crosses over the sacroiliac joint, and when it goes into spasm it can create sacroiliac joint discomfort, causing pain in the low back and hip. Second, when in spasm, the piriformis can entrap the sciatic nerve. The sciatic nerve is the major nerve supplying the muscles for the entire leg all the way to the bottom of the foot. If the piriformis muscle entraps the sciatic nerve, pain may radiate down the athlete's leg. Third, the piriformis muscle may be strained or develop trigger points within the muscle, which will create pain around the sacrum or the hip.

Massage strokes used for treating the six deep lateral rotators muscles are petrissage, compression strokes, stripping strokes, direct pressure, cross-fiber friction, and compression strokes to finish. The athlete lies facedown with a bolster under the ankles. (The athlete may leave her clothing on for these treatments.) The trainer applies petrissage to the hip on the side where the athlete is experiencing discomfort. Petrissage should be applied to the posterior hip around the hip joint for 30 seconds. Next, stripping strokes are applied from the hip to the sacrum 10 times. When performing the stripping strokes, the trainer can stop at any tender areas and hold direct pressure for 8 to 12 seconds until the tenderness subsides. After applying stripping and direct pressure to the lateral rotators, the trainer applies cross-fiber friction to the edge of the sacrum and the hip and then finishes the massage treatment with compression strokes.

To finish the treatment, stretches should be applied to the six deep lateral rotator muscles. With the athlete in the facedown position, the trainer lifts the lower leg to 90 degrees. The trainer should have one hand on the athlete's hip and the other hand around the athlete's ankle. The trainer then rotates the athlete's hip away from the body until it is stretched, holds the hip in the stretched position for two seconds, and then releases. The hip should be stretched eight times.

If residual soreness is still present, a topical analgesic can be applied to the hip three times a day. This treatment may be applied every other day until the condition improves.

Back

Almost all athletes love to have their back massaged. The erector spinae muscles, the powerful muscles along either side of the spine, hold the body erect. These muscles are often sore and should be targeted during sport massage. Common movements like running, jumping, throwing, and swinging motions can cause back discomfort. Running and jumping are more likely to cause low-back discomfort, and throwing and swinging motions can cause midback and upper back discomfort. Rotating motions of the back require the spine to twist. If muscles of the back become tight or are in spasm, the quick forceful rotations of the spine can create back discomfort.

Massage strokes used for treating the back muscles are compressive effleurage, circular friction, petrissage, compression strokes, direct pressure, and compressive effleurage to finish. The athlete lies facedown with the face in the face cradle and a bolster under the ankles. The massage begins with long effleurage strokes along the spine from the shoulders down the back to the sacrum. The trainer stands at the head of the table, applies massage lubricant to her or his hands, and spreads the lubricant down the back while performing 10 compressive effleurage strokes. The trainer moves to the side of the table and applies circular friction to the opposite side of the athlete's back from the shoulder to the hip. Next, petrissage is applied from the hip to the shoulder on the same side three times. The trainer then applies compression strokes three times to the muscles on the same side along the spine from the low back up the spine to the base of the neck. The application of circular friction, petrissage, and compression is repeated on the other side of the back. The trainer then applies direct pressure along each side of the spine three times, making sure to apply the pressure to the athlete's comfort level. While performing direct pressure, the trainer can stop at any tender areas and hold direct pressure on them for 8 to 12 seconds. The massage treatment should end with 10 compressive effleurage strokes down the back for comfort.

To finish the treatment for the back, the athlete should perform ranges of motion. The athlete should stand up and bend forward, then backward, then side to side, and then rotate to both sides, performing these motions eight times. If residual soreness is still present in the back muscles, a topical analgesic can be applied to the back. The analgesic can be applied three times a day every other day until the condition improves.

Shoulders

The upper trapezius, the area between the neck and shoulder, is a primary target of the shoulder for sport massage. The upper trapezius is the muscle in the body most likely to develop trigger points. Trigger points are localized areas of tenderness in the bellies of muscles that refer pain when compressed. The trapezius muscles elevate the shoulder and assists movement of the neck. Sports that require throwing motions of the shoulder or that involve swinging a racket, club, or bat place stress on the upper trapezius.

Massage strokes used for treating the upper shoulder are compressive effleurage, circular friction, petrissage, compression strokes, direct pressure, and compressive effleurage to finish. The upper shoulder treatment begins with the athlete lying facedown with a bolster under the ankles. The trainer applies a small amount of Prossage Heat to the hands and performs compressive effleurage strokes to the top of one shoulder, moving from compressive effleurage strokes to circular friction of the shoulder for 30 seconds. After applying circular friction, the trainer applies petrissage from the shoulder to the base of neck three times and applies compression strokes along the top of the shoulder three times. The trainer then gently pinches the upper trapezius muscle from the shoulder to the base of the neck, making sure that the pressure is tolerable to the athlete. Next, direct pressure is applied along the top of the shoulder three times. The upper shoulder massage ends with 10 compressive effleurage strokes. Strokes are repeated to the opposite shoulder.

To finish the treatment for the upper shoulder, the athlete performs shoulder shrugs. The athlete should stand up and tighten the muscles across the top of the shoulder by bringing the shoulders up toward the ears and holding in the elevated position for eight seconds. The athlete should perform shoulder shrugs eight times. If residual soreness is still present in the upper shoulder muscles, a topical analgesic can be applied three times a day. This treatment may be applied every other day until the condition improves.

Forearms

After the shoulders, the next most common area of complaint is the forearms. The powerful forearm muscles control the wrist and hand. Motions like throwing a ball and swinging a racket or club are common causes of forearm muscle soreness. Overuse discomfort in this area can cause pain at the inside or outside of the elbow, known as tennis or golfer's elbow.

Massage strokes used for treating the forearm are compressive effleurage, compression strokes, stripping strokes, direct pressure, cross-fiber friction, and compressive effleurage to finish.

The trainer starts the massage treatment for the forearms by having the athlete lie faceup on the massage table with the arms by the sides and the palms facing downward. A bolster should be under the athlete's knees. The trainer applies a small portion of Prossage Heat to his hands and begins the forearm treatment with compressive effleurage from the wrist to the elbow 10 times. Next are compression strokes from the elbow to the wrist three times. Stripping strokes are then performed from the wrist to the elbow three times. When tender spots are encountered during the application of stripping strokes, direct pressure can be applied for 8 to 12 seconds. After stripping strokes and direct pressure have been applied, cross-fiber friction is applied at the elbow for 30 seconds. The athlete should provide feedback about the amount of pressure used. The forearm massage treatment ends with the application of compressive effleurage 10 times from the wrist to the elbow. The preceding techniques are repeated on the other side of the forearms.

To finish the treatment for the forearm, the athlete moves the wrist backward until it stops, holds for two seconds, and then releases. The athlete then moves the wrist forward until it stops, holds for two seconds, and then releases. The athlete should perform the back-and-forth movements eight times.

TREATMENTS FOR SPECIFIC SPORTS

This section addresses applications of sport massage for some common conditions in specific sports. Each sport section provides an overview of the physical movements involved and discusses the conditions that commonly occur from repetition of the movements of that sport. For each sport, the most common conditions specific to that sport and treatments for the conditions are discussed. (Sports such as football, baseball, basketball, and soccer that involve running create stresses on the same areas of the athlete's body. So, some of the conditions listed under one sport may occur in other sports as well.)

According to estimates, there are over 75 million runners in the United States. Runners come in all shapes and sizes and with different abilities, but they all have to propel their bodies in an upright position against gravity and wind. Although running is a full-body activity, it places great stress on the lower extremities. The biomechanics of running always starts with the foot strike. As the foot strikes, so goes the rest of the body. A runner with continual foot, ankle, calf, and knee pain might want to have his or her feet checked to see whether orthotics might improve biomechanics. Orthotics are inserts designed to support the arches of the foot during walking or running. Podiatrists and chiropractors often screen athletes for proper foot and ankle function. Two of the most common causes of problems for runners are running shoes that fit improperly and poor biomechanics of the foot and ankle.

JOGGER'S HEEL

The first part of the foot to strike the ground is the lateral heel, making it prone to a pounding punishment. This continual impact may cause the heel pad to become inflamed and sore to the touch. During a run, this pain can increase to the point that a runner cannot continue. A mild case is referred to as jogger's heel. If it goes untreated, the runner can develop heel spurs. Jogger's heel is pain felt in the heel pad of the foot that is aggravating but tolerable when walking or running. Heel spurs are calcium formations that form on the bottom of the heel and can become so intense that walking is difficult. Heel spurs may require surgical intervention.

Treatment

Massage of the runner's foot begins with the athlete lying in the facedown position with a bolster under the ankles. The trainer applies a few drops of Prossage Heat to the bottom of the runner's foot and uses compressive effleurage strokes 10 times. Stripping strokes are then applied three times from the ball of the foot to the heel from the inside of the foot to the outside. The trainer can locate any tender areas on the heel pad by pushing the heel pad with the thumbs. Holding direct pressure on the tender area for two to four seconds three times may reduce the discomfort. After the discomfort has lessened, gentle cross-fiber friction is applied to free up any remaining tenderness remaining in the pad.

BUNIONS

When a runner's weight transfers from the heel to the front of the foot, the big toe bears most of the stress. A big toe that does not project straight forward can lead to the formation of bunions. Bunions are bony protuberances that form at the base of the big toe. The three common causes of the formation of bunions are wearing pointed shoes (high heels), loss of proper arch structure, and heredity. Athletes with this condition often have a family history of bunions.

Treatment

After massaging the bottom of the foot, the trainer applies massage to the big toe with the finger and thumb for 30 seconds. After massage has been applied, the trainer stretches the big toe away from the midline of the foot 30 times using the thumb and index finger. This movement may be uncomfortable to the athlete because the joint may be red, swollen, and calcified, so the movement should be gentle at the beginning.

If residual soreness is still present in the heel and bunion, the whole foot should be soaked in cool water for 20 minutes. After the foot is dried off, topical analgesic can be applied. This treatment may be applied three times a day every other day until the condition improves.

CYCLING

About 87 million Americans ride bicycles. Many people enjoy cycling because it is an inexpensive form of exercise that helps them stay healthy and fit. Some athletes choose cycling because it is not jarring to the body. Even so, the physical demands of cycling on the bodies of serious cyclists can be exhausting. In the riding position the cyclist's upper body is hunched forward, the head is held up in the straightforward position, and the arms are outstretched in front. The shoes are clipped into toe clips, and the legs are constantly churning. Cycling becomes especially difficult when riding up hills or pedaling against strong winds.

The legs and hips are the prime area of stress in cycling. The legs of a cyclist undergo constant stress. The constant pedaling leads to fatigue of the quadriceps, the hamstring, and the calf muscles. As the leg muscles fatigue, they often begin to spasm and cramp. An unconditioned cyclist usually ends the ride at this point. Well-conditioned riders drink fluid and push through the pain. Often, the constant stress from the legs will start to affect both the front and side of the knee.

CHONDROMALACIA PATELLA

Chondromalacia patella is an irritation of the knee caused by the quadriceps muscles compressing the patella (kneecap) against the end of the femur. The kneecap has a layer of smooth cartilage on its undersurface that is vulnerable to wear from constant pressure. The cartilage of the patella normally glides effortlessly over the knee joint. The pressure from the thigh muscles pushing the patella against cartilage in the knee can irritate the cartilage surface.

Treatment

The athlete lies faceup on the massage table with a bolster under the knees. The trainer applies a small amount of lubricant over the thigh muscles using compressive effleurage strokes 10 times. Petrissage strokes are then applied to the inside, top, and outside of the thigh, with three passes over each area. Next, compression strokes are applied along the same three areas of the thigh three times. The trainer then applies stripping strokes in the same three areas. If tender areas are encountered, the trainer stops and holds for two to four seconds, applying direct pressure three times. The next step is to apply a few drops of Prossage Heat and friction on the top, bottom, sides, and ligament of the patella with the thumb for two minutes. The trainer then applies broadening strokes to the thigh from the hip to the knee three times and finishes the massage with compressive effleurage strokes from just below the knee to the top of the hip.

To finish the treatment, stretches should be applied to the quadriceps muscles. The athlete turns to the side-lying position on the massage table and flexes the bottom knee to the waist. The athlete holds the ankle of the top leg, brings the knee of the top leg to the chest, and extends the top knee until it is in a straight line with the rest of the body. The athlete should hold the stretch for two seconds and then bring the top knee back to the chest. A trainer may assist this stretch. As the athlete brings the knee back, the trainer pushes in on the athlete's hip and gently pulls the knee back. The stretch should be performed eight times. If residual soreness is still present in the knee, an ice pack can be applied for 20 minutes. Topical analgesic can then be applied to the knee three times a day every other day until the condition improves.

ILIOTIBIAL BAND SYNDROME

Iliotibial band syndrome is common injury of the thigh from activities like running and cycling. The iliotibial band is a thick fibrous tendon that runs down the outside of the thigh. The origin of the iliotibial band is from two muscles that attach to the hip. In the front lateral part of the hip is a muscle called tensor fascia lata, and in back is the large gluteus maximus insert onto the upper part of the iliotibial band. The iliotibial band then travels down the side of the thigh and inserts across the knee at the lateral condyle of the tibia. The function of the band is to provide support for the outside of the knee during walking and running. In cycling, the muscles of the thigh become engorged with blood and expand. This expansion of the thigh muscles creates extra pressure on the band running down the outside of the thigh. As the knee bends and straightens during the pedaling motion, the iliotibial band flips over a bony prominence just above the knee called the lateral epicondyle of the femur. This constant flipping of the band starts to inflame the band, causing pain and discomfort.

Treatment

The treatment starts with the athlete lying faceup on the massage table with a bolster under the knees. The trainer applies a small amount of lubricant over the thigh muscles with compressive effleurage strokes 10 times. Compression strokes are then applied to the top and outside of the thigh three times. Next, stripping strokes are applied along the outside area of the thigh. If the trainer encounters tender areas when applying the stripping strokes, she can stop and apply direct pressure for two to four seconds. A few drops of Prossage Heat can be applied to the area just above the knee on the outside, often the location of the most tender area of iliotibial band syndrome. When applying friction, the trainer should ask for feedback from the athlete. The friction technique should be done gently, and the discomfort in the area should go from sharp to dull. Friction should be applied to the area for 15 seconds three times, using a rest period of a minute after each. The massage ends with compressive effleurage strokes from just below the knee to the top of the hip.

To finish the treatment, stretches should be applied to the iliotibial band. The athlete lies on the back and performs a straight leg raise with the leg that has the iliotibial band syndrome while keeping the knee locked. The straight leg is brought across the athlete's body as far as it will stretch and held for two seconds. A trainer may assist with this stretch. As the athlete brings the leg across the body, the trainer places one hand on the hip being stretched and uses the other hand to assist the athlete in bringing the leg across the body. The athlete then returns the leg to the resting position on the table. The stretch should be performed eight times. If residual soreness is still present in the knee, an ice pack can be applied for 20 minutes. After the ice pack application is complete, topical analgesic is applied to the knee three times a day. This treatment may be applied every other day until the condition improves.

SWIMMING

Swimming is a popular sport in the United States. Competition typically starts at a young age. Many athletes believe that swimming is one of the best workouts for the body because it works all the major muscle groups at the same time. As the swimmer propels the body through the water, the water can create up to 10 times the resistance of air. As a workout, swimming is one of the safest because the body is submerged in water where the motions do not create the pressure on the joints and muscles that other sports can. Another advantage of swimming is that the athlete can choose to specialize in the stroke that feels best for her or his body. Freestyle is the most popular stroke, followed by breaststroke, backstroke, and the butterfly. With swimming, practicing often and for long periods increases the possibility of incurring repetitive use injuries.

SWIMMER'S SHOULDER

Swimmer's shoulder is an injury that refers to rotator cuff inflammation, soreness, and possibly tendinitis of the shoulder. It is common in freestyle, backstroke, and butterfly swimmers because these strokes require the swimmer to reach out with the arms while performing the strokes. A competitive college swimmer may rotate the shoulder up to one million times in a year.

The three muscles of the back of the shoulder are referred to as the rotator cuff muscles: supraspinatus on top, infraspinatus in the middle, and teres minor along the outside border. The three rotator cuff muscles attach to the back of the upper arm at a bump called the greater tuberosity of the humerus. During a rotation of the shoulder, there is not much space between the head of the humerus (upper arm bone) and the acromion (shoulder blade). The rotator cuff muscles can be pinched between the two bones, causing microtrauma to the tendons and bellies of the muscles, which results in inflammation and soreness in the shoulder

Treatment

The treatment starts with the athlete lying facedown with the arms by the side and a bolster under the ankles. The trainer adds lubricant to the hands and applies circular friction to the top and back of the shoulder for 30 seconds. Next, petrissage is applied to the top and outside of the shoulder for three passes. Compression of the top, outside, and back of the shoulder follows. Stripping strokes are then applied from the shoulder to the scapula along these muscles three times. Where tender spots are located, direct pressure can be held for two to four seconds. The trainer places a few drops of Prossage Heat on the back upper part of the shoulder and performs cross-fiber friction to the greater tuberosity of the humerus for 30 seconds three times with a 1-minute rest after each application. The discomfort from the cross-fiber friction applied to the greater tuberosity should always go from sharp to dull. The trainer finishes the massage of the top and back of the shoulder with compressive effleurage 10 times.

To finish the treatment, the athlete moves the shoulder through its normal range of motion. The athlete starts by moving the arm from the side in an arc until it is straight up in the air eight times. Next, the athlete brings the arm to shoulder height with the elbow bent at 90 degrees and performs internal and external rotation of the shoulder eight times. If residual soreness is still present in the shoulder, an ice pack should be applied for 20 minutes. A topical analgesic can be applied to the shoulder three times a day on alternate days until the condition improves.

SWIMMER'S KNEE

Swimmer's knee is caused by the whip kick used while performing the breaststroke. This kick takes the knee from flexion to extension and causes stress to the medial collateral ligament of the knee. The medial collateral ligament (sometimes referred to as the tibial collateral ligament) holds the upper and lower leg bones together. As the knee moves from flexion to extension, the stress on the ligament increases, causing microtrauma to the ligament, which in turn causes inflammation and soreness in the medial side of the knee.

Treatment

The athlete starts in the face-up position with a bolster under the knees. Lubricant is applied with compressive effleurage to the knee 10 times. Petrissage is then applied to the inside of the leg from the calf to the inner thigh. The medial collateral ligament is located by pressing along the inside of the knee between the lower leg and the thigh. The trainer must be careful because the ligament could be quite tender. He or she adds a few drops of Prossage Heat to the area and performs gentle cross-fiber friction on the ligament for 30 seconds with a 1-minute rest period between applications. Discomfort should always move from sharp to dull during the application. The massage concludes with application of compressive effleurage to the knee 10 times.

The trainer finishes the treatment by having the athlete move the knee through its normal range of motion by flexing and extending the knee eight times. The athlete should stand up and perform squats eight times as long as the motion does not cause discomfort. If residual soreness is still present in the knee, an ice pack can be applied for 20 minutes. After the ice pack application, topical analgesic is applied to the knee. The analgesic should be applied three times a day every other day until the condition improves.

FOOTBALL

From pee wee to professional, athletes of all ages love to play football. All kinds of athletes play football, including linemen with large, tall, and strong bodies to running backs and receivers with fast, tough, and strong bodies. These big guys run at each other as hard as they can. Football is one of the roughest contact sports in the world. Even with protective equipment like helmets and shoulder pads, injuries are inevitable because the instant the football is snapped, the feet push off and the shoulders slam into other players.

TURF TOE

Turf toe gets its name from an injury to the big toe that is caused by the front of the foot being caught on hard artificial playing surfaces. At awkward moments, the player's foot is caught and the toes are bent backward, straining the big toe, the joint capsule, and its ligaments. The purpose of the massage treatment is to relieve some of the pain and discomfort of the injury and to aid in improving range of motion and function. In the early stages of injury, it is difficult for the athlete to place weight on the injured foot. The immediate treatment is to reduce inflammation by soaking the foot in cold water. After the acute inflammatory response has subsided, massage treatment may be administered.

Treatment

The treatment starts with the athlete lying faceup with a bolster under the knees. The trainer applies massage lubricant to the top and bottom of the foot using compressive effleurage 10 times. Next, compression strokes are applied to the inside and bottom of the foot three times. The trainer then applies stripping strokes along the side and bottom of the foot three times, stopping at any tender areas and holding for two to four seconds. Prossage Heat is then placed on the ball of the foot and big toe, and friction is applied three times with the finger and thumb for 30 seconds with a rest of 1 minute after each application. The massage ends with compressive effleurage strokes on the top and bottom of the foot 10 times.

To finish the treatment, the athlete flexes and extends the big toe at the end of each movement. The trainer gently stretches the toe, being careful not to push the big toe backward with too much force. The athlete should provide feedback about the level of discomfort. If residual soreness is still present in the foot and big toe, they should be soaked in cold water for 20 minutes. After the foot is dried off, topical analgesic is applied to the foot and big toe. This treatment can be applied three times a day every other day until the condition improves.

CERVICAL STINGER

A cervical stinger (or burner) is a nerve injury of the neck and shoulder. Estimates are that half of all high school and college football players have experienced at least one stinger or burner. A football player who tackles another player often drops one shoulder and drives it into the player being tackled. The force of the collision forces the tackler's shoulder down and the head back. This movement can stretch the network of nerves (known as the brachial plexus) traveling through the shoulder. When the nerves are stretched, a burning or stinging sensation travels down the arm and can leave the arm numb and weak. The symptoms can last for a few minutes to months, depending on severity. Sport massage is not intended to cure stingers or burners. The goal of the treatment is to reduce discomfort in the neck, shoulder, and arm.

Treatment

To start, the athlete lies facedown with the head in a face cradle and a bolster under the ankles. The arms are at the sides with the hands palm up. Lubricant is applied with compressive effleurage from the wrist to the shoulder. Compression strokes to the forearm and back of the upper arm follow. Next, stripping strokes are applied to the forearm and then the back of the upper arm three times. When applying stripping strokes, the trainer should stop on any tender areas and hold for two to four seconds. Compressive effleurage strokes are then applied from the arm to the back of the neck. Next, Prossage Heat is applied with petrissage along the top of the shoulder and the back of the neck three times. The trainer then applies stripping strokes along the top of the shoulder and the back of the neck, stopping at any tender areas and holding direct pressure for two to four seconds. Petrissage is then applied along the top of the shoulder and the back of the neck. The massage treatment ends with compressive effleurage from the wrist to the back of the neck.

To finish the treatment, the athlete flexes and extends the neck. At the end of each movement, the trainer may provide gentle stretching. The athlete then moves the neck from side to side, and gentle stretching can be used at the end of each movement. The trainer must be careful not to push the neck with too much force when stretching the neck from side to side. Asking the athlete for feedback about the level of discomfort is useful. If residual soreness is still present in the neck and shoulder, an ice pack should be applied for 20 minutes. Topical analgesic should then be used on the shoulder and neck. The analgesic should be applied three times a day every other day until the condition improves.

Baseball has been called America's pastime since the 19th century because it was the most widely played sport in the United States. Baseball today is currently the second most popular sport in the United States following football. Baseball can be played for many years if the body can withstand the physical demands. The throwing motion in baseball can stress the upper extremity to the point that continuing to play is difficult.

ROTATOR CUFF SORENESS

The shoulder is prone to injuries because of muscular imbalances across the shoulder joint. In the throwing motion the arm moves from external rotation into medial rotation with considerable force. The five medial rotator muscles are the anterior deltoid, pectoralis major, latissimus dorsi, teres major, and subscapularis. The three lateral rotator muscles are the posterior deltoid, infraspinatus, and teres minor. The medial rotator muscles are stronger and more flexible than the external rotators. This muscular imbalance is often a contributing factor to rotator cuff soreness.

Treatment

The athlete lies facedown on the massage table with a bolster under the ankles. The trainer applies massage lubricant with effleurage strokes to the top and back of the shoulder 10 times and then applies circular friction to the top and back of the shoulder for 30 seconds. Petrissage is then applied to the top and side of the shoulder three times. Next, compression is applied to the top and back of the shoulder three times. The trainer then applies Prossage Heat and stripping strokes along the top, middle, and edge of the shoulder blade three times, stopping at any tender areas and holding for two to four seconds. The trainer applies friction to the arm at the back of the shoulder. The massage may end with compressive effleurage of the shoulder 10 times.

To finish the shoulder treatment, the athlete sits up and raises the arm to shoulder height with the elbow flexed to 90 degrees. The athlete rotates the shoulder in internal rotation, gently stretches for two seconds, and then releases. The athlete then rotates the shoulder in external rotation, gently stretches for two seconds, and then releases. Internal and external rotation should be performed eight times. If residual soreness is still present in the shoulder, an ice pack should be used for 20 minutes. Topical analgesic should then be applied to the shoulder and neck three times a day. This treatment can be applied every other day until the condition improves.

MEDIAL ELBOW TENDINITIS

The most common tendons affected by the throwing motion in the elbow are on the inside or medial part of the elbow. Two groups of muscles originate at the medial epicondyle of the elbow: the wrist flexors, which bend the wrist down toward the ground, and the forearm pronator, which rotates the palm from the palm-up to the palm-down position. The throwing motion can irritate the muscles and tendons, creating inflammation and soreness. The first part of the treatment is always directed at reducing the acute inflammation before massage can begin.

Treatment

The athlete lies faceup on the massage table with a bolster under knees, the arms at the sides, and the palms facing up. The trainer applies lubricant to the forearm from the wrist to the elbow using compressive effleurage 10 times. Compression strokes from the elbow to the wrist are then applied three times. Next, stripping strokes are applied from the wrist to the inside of the elbow three times. If any tender spots are located, the trainer should apply direct pressure and hold for 12 seconds. Next, Prossage Heat is applied to the inside of the elbow and gentle cross-fiber friction is applied there for 30 seconds. After a 1-minute rest, cross-fiber friction is used again for 30 seconds. The massage treatment ends with the application of compressive effleurage 10 times.

To finish the elbow treatment, the athlete moves the wrist in flexion and extension and holds in each position for two seconds. He performs each stretch eight times. The athlete then moves the wrist to palm-up position and then palm-down position and holds in each position for two seconds. He performs each stretch eight times.

BASKETBALL

James Naismith, a teacher at a YMCA in Springfield, Massachusetts, is credited with inventing the game of basketball in 1891. From its early beginning, it has grown into the college "March Madness" championship and the NBA championship. Basketball players must possess speed, strength, and endurance. An explosive first step allows basketball players to drive past or through a defensive player to score. Players must be able to go from standing still to running full speed quickly. They must have the strength to jump high enough to dunk a basketball, and they need sufficient endurance to do it the entire game and over a long season. When they jump to shoot or dunk a basketball, they must land on their feet in a controlled motion. This full-speed running, jumping, and landing is all done on a hard wooden floor, which makes the action punishing to the body.

JUMPER'S KNEE

Jumper's knee is an overuse condition that causes the patellar ligament of the knee to become irritated and inflamed. The patellar ligament connects the kneecap to the shinbone. The big, powerful quadriceps muscles of the leg anterior attach to the top of the patella. The patellar ligament connects the bottom of the patella to the shin. When the quadriceps muscles contract, the thigh straightens the leg in jumping to propel the athlete off the ground. The quadriceps muscles also help stabilize the knee when the athlete lands after jumping. Pressure placed on the ligament is usually painful, and jumping or kneeling can aggravate the condition.

Treatment

The athlete starts in face-up position with a bolster under the knees. The trainer applies massage lubricant to the thigh using compressive effleurage from the knee to the hip 10 times. Petrissage strokes are then applied to the inside, top, and outside of the thigh three times. Next, compression strokes are applied to the outside, top, and inside of the thigh three times. The trainer then applies stripping strokes along the outside, top, and inside of the thigh three times, stopping at any tender points and holding for two to four seconds. Next, Prossage Heat is applied to the anterior knee. The trainer uses friction on the top, sides, and bottom of the patella for 30 seconds three times with a 1-minute rest between applications. The cross-fiber friction should be adjusted to the athlete's comfort level. The final massage technique is the application of compressive effleurage from the knee to the hip 10 times.

To finish the treatment, stretches should be applied to the quadriceps muscles. The athlete turns to the side-lying position on the massage table and flexes the bottom knee to the waist. She holds the ankle of the top leg, brings the knee of the top leg to the chest, extends the top knee until it is in a straight line with the rest of the body, holds the stretch for two seconds, and then brings the top knee back to the chest. The athlete should perform the stretch eight times. If residual soreness is still present in the knee, an ice pack can be applied for 20 minutes. After the ice pack application, topical analgesic can be applied to the knee. The analgesic can be applied three times a day every other day until the condition improves.

SPRAINED ANKLE

Jumping is hard not only on the knee but also on the ankle. Basketball players can land awkwardly after jumping. Ankle sprains occur when the foot turns or twists, which often happens when a player jumps and lands on another player's foot. If the foot lands awkwardly with enough force, ligaments that hold the ankle together can stretch beyond their normal range of motion. The amount of pain that an athlete experiences from a sprained ankle usually depends on the amount of damage that occurred. Walking often becomes difficult because of the amount of pain and swelling. Obtaining a proper medical diagnosis is important.

Treatment

The athlete lies facedown on the massage table with a bolster under the ankles. The trainer lifts the athlete's lower leg to 90 degrees and applies massage lubricant to the foot and ankle. The athlete then points the foot toward the ceiling. The trainer places both hands around the foot and ankle. As the athlete moves the foot toward the table, the trainer pulls down with both hands around the ankle. This technique helps reduce swelling in the ankle after the acute stage of injury has subsided (48 to 72 hours after the injury). The technique is performed 10 times. With the leg back on the table, Prossage Heat is applied to the outside of the ankle. Gentle cross-fiber friction is applied around the bottom of the outside ankle bone (lateral malleolus). The ligament in the anterior lateral aspect of the ankle, called the anterior talofibular ligament, is the ligament most often sprained in the ankle. Gentle cross-fiber friction can be applied three times for 30 seconds with a 1-minute rest between applications. The pressure should be adjusted to the athlete's comfort level.

To finish the treatment, stretches should be applied to the ankle. The athlete lies face up on the table, gently points the foot down toward the table, and then pulls the foot up toward the head. The trainer may assist with these stretches by providing a gentle stretch at the end of each motion. The ankle is gently stretched for two seconds in each position and this is performed eight times. If residual soreness is still present in the ankle, it should be soaked in cold water for 20 minutes. After the ankle is dried off, topical analgesic can be applied to the knee. Application can be made three times a day every other day until the condition improves.

Soccer is played in almost every country in the world. More than 240 million people play soccer worldwide. Soccer players are well-conditioned athletes. Because they must run throughout most of the game, players need great endurance, speed, flexibility, and stamina. A soccer player may run up to 7 miles (11 km) in a single game. Soccer players are usually trim because of the intense amount of energy expended playing the game. Because soccer requires almost constant running, the ankles, knees, and hips of soccer players are common sites of soreness. It is a good thing that soccer is played on grass because otherwise considerably more injuries would occur. Soccer players often use the body or head to direct the soccer ball. Banging the ball with the head can lead to sore neck muscles.

HAMSTRING STRAINS

Hamstring strains are often referred to as pulled hamstrings. A hamstring strain is the most common injury to the thigh. When running, the quadriceps muscles move the thigh forward and the hamstrings pull the thigh backward. The quadriceps muscles on the front of the thigh are always stronger than the hamstrings in the back of the thigh. If the hamstrings become tight, the force of the quadriceps' contraction can overpower the hamstrings and pull or strain them. Hamstring strains are graded according to severity. First-degree strains are the mildest, second-degree strains are more severe, and third-degree strains are the most severe. Higher degrees of strain cause greater pain, muscle spasm, and swelling.

Treatment

The treatment starts with the athlete lying facedown on the table with a bolster under the ankles. The trainer applies massage lubricant with compressive effleurage strokes on the back of the thigh 10 times. Petrissage is then applied to the back of the thigh from the hip to the knee three times. Next, Prossage Heat and stripping strokes are applied from the outside of the back of the knee up the thigh to the center of the back of the thigh. While performing the stripping strokes, the trainer should stop at any tender points and hold for two to four seconds. He should have the athlete raise the leg to 90 degrees and hold the ankle. The athlete should pull the ankle toward the hip but not let the lower leg move. If tenderness is experienced in the hamstring muscle with this maneuver, the athlete should touch the area of tenderness. The trainer should compress the area while moving the athlete's leg back and forth. Next, gentle cross-fiber friction can be applied to the tender area for 30 seconds three times with a 1-minute rest between applications. The trainer may finish the massage with compressive effleurage to the back of the thigh from the knee to the hip 10 times.

To finish the treatment, stretches should be applied to the hamstrings. The athlete lies faceup on the massage table, locks the knee, and performs a straight leg raise. Wherever the leg stops, the trainer holds the thigh while the athlete flexes the knee. The trainer helps the athlete straighten the leg, holds for two seconds, and then releases. The bent-knee hamstring stretch should be performed eight times. The athlete returns the leg to resting position on the massage table and then performs a straight leg raise with the knee locked. At the end of the motion, the trainer gently stretches the athlete's straight leg toward the head for two seconds and then returns the leg to resting position. The straight leg raise is performed eight times. If residual soreness is still present in the hamstrings, an ice pack can be applied for 20 minutes. A topical analgesic can then be applied to the knee three times a day on alternate days until the condition improves.

NECK STRAINS

Neck strains are a partial tearing of the neck muscles. In soccer, neck injuries can occur when the player uses the head to strike the ball. As the soccer ball approaches, the player must tighten the neck muscles before heading the ball. The speed and weight of the ball can whip the head and neck if the neck muscles are not tightened before contact. The amount of soreness in the neck after heading the ball is often a signal of the severity of the injury.

Treatment

The athlete starts in facedown position with the face in a face cradle and a bolster under the ankles. The trainer applies massage lubricant with effleurage strokes from the neck to the midback 10 times. Petrissage is then applied to the neck and upper shoulders three times. Next, stripping strokes are applied from the head to the base of the neck three times. While performing the stripping strokes, the trainer can stop at any tender points and hold for two to four seconds. Gentle cross-fiber friction with Prossage Heat is then applied along the back of the base of the skull for 30 seconds three times with a 1-minute rest after each application. The trainer finishes the massage treatment with compressive effleurage from the head to midback 10 times.

To finish the treatment, stretches should be applied to the athlete's neck. The athlete lies in the face-up position. As the athlete raises the head toward the chest, the trainer gently pushes the back of the athlete's head forward and holds for two seconds. The stretch should be performed eight times. Next, the athlete tilts the head sideways to touch the ear to the shoulder, and the trainer gently pushes for two seconds. Side-bending stretches should be performed eight times on each side of neck. Finally, the athlete rotates the head to the shoulder, and the trainer gently stretches the head in rotation and holds for two seconds. Neck rotations should be performed eight times to each shoulder. If residual soreness is still present in the neck, an ice pack can be applied for 20 minutes. After the ice pack application, topical analgesic can be applied to the neck three times a day. This treatment may be applied every other day until the condition improves.

GOLF

The game of golf may have been invented more than 2,000 years ago by shepherds who used their curved staffs to hit stones. A more formal version of the game emerged in Scotland over 1,000 years ago. Today, roughly 26 million people play golf every year in the United States alone. Pro golfers make the game look easy: They have a club, and they swing at a ball. How difficult can that be? But in reality, golf is a difficult game to learn. The golf swing is unlike any other swing in sport. The golf stance, grip, body rotation, arm swing, and speed of the stroke make it one of the most difficult maneuvers in sports. In fact, millions of dollars are spent each year on golf lessons and clubs in an attempt to perfect the swing.

Most people are not strong enough or flexible enough in the midbody area to perform a proper swing. As a result, they cannot maintain proper position or rotate the midbody, so they compensate with arm swing. A golf swing generated primarily from arm swing is usually not effective. As with pitching a baseball, the power of a golf swing is generated from the feet up. The feet push against the ground, and a ripple of muscle contractions flows from the feet to the hips through the trunk and out the arms. The sum of all the muscle contractions through the body creates the power of the swing. Anything that disrupts the smooth flow of muscle contractions distorts the swing.

BACK PAIN

The golf swing puts a great deal of stress on the low back, and even bending over to putt the golf ball is stressful to the lower back. Low-back pain is the most common problem encountered by golfers today. Rotation of the spine should take place mostly in the neck with a little help from the mid- and upper back. Because of the design of the vertebral joints, the lower back, or lumbar area of the back, was not meant to twist. The force of the golf swing can irritate the low back, causing the muscles to go into spasm.

Treatment

The athlete lies in the facedown position with the face in a face cradle and a bolster under the ankles. Massage lubricant is applied with 10 compressive effleurage strokes to the low back. Compression strokes are then applied on each side of the spine three times. Next, the trainer applies stripping strokes along each side of spine, stopping at any tender points and holding for four seconds. Prossage Heat is then applied to the low-back area. The trainer applies cross-fiber friction to the muscles of the low back and the top of the hips for 30 seconds three times with a rest of 1 minute after each application. The massage treatment ends with compressive effleurage strokes 10 times in the low back.

To finish the treatment, stretches should be applied to the athlete's lower back. The athlete lies on the massage table in the face-up position. The athlete brings one knee to the chest, and the trainer gently pushes the knee toward the chest to stretch the lower back. The stretched position should be held for two seconds and performed eight times. The athlete may then perform the straight leg raise eight times on each leg, stretching the leg for two seconds. If residual soreness is still present in the low back, an ice pack can be applied for 20 minutes. A topical analgesic can be applied to the lower back three times a day every other day until the condition improves.

GOLFER'S ELBOW

Golfer's elbow, or medial epicondylitis, is pain and inflammation that occurs on the inside of the elbow. The most common cause of golfer's elbow is overuse. Tendons at the end of the forearm muscles that attach to the medial epicondyle can become injured because of a single violent action like swinging a golf club into the ground or because of the repetitive stress of the golf swing.

Treatment

To start, the athlete lies faceup on the massage table with a bolster under the knees, the arms at the sides, and the palms facing up. The trainer applies lubricant to the forearm from the wrist to the elbow using compressive effleurage 10 times. Compression strokes are then applied from the elbow to the wrist three times. Next, the trainer applies stripping strokes from the wrist to the inside of the elbow three times. If the trainer locates any tender spots while applying stripping strokes, she or he should apply direct pressure and hold for two to four seconds. Next, the trainer applies Prossage Heat to the inside of the elbow and gently applies cross-fiber friction to that area three times for 30 seconds with a rest of 1 minute after each application. The massage treatment ends with the application of compressive effleurage 10 times.

To finish the elbow treatment, the athlete moves the wrist in flexion and extension, holding in each position for two seconds and performing the action eight times. The athlete moves the wrist to the palm-up position and then the palm-down position, holding each position for two seconds and performing the stretch eight times. If residual soreness is still present at the medial elbow, an ice pack can be applied for 20 minutes. After the ice treatment, topical analgesic is applied to the medial elbow. The analgesic can be applied three times a day on alternate days until the condition improves.

TENNIS

In 1873 a Welshman named Major Walter Wingfield introduced the game of lawn tennis (although he called it Sphairistike, apparently based on the Greek word for playing ball), which eventually became the modern game of tennis. Tennis players today must have catlike reflexes to be able to move forward, backward, and side to side as needed to meet the ball. The speed of the game requires players to anticipate where the tennis ball is going before it is hit. Like baseball players at bat, tennis players must swing and return serves coming at them at high speeds. The head of a tennis racket is much bigger than the width of a baseball bat, but returning a serve is no easier than hitting a baseball. The eye–hand coordination of a tennis player is incredible. The player must position his or her body and the tennis racket in the right place before the ball arrives to have any chance of returning a serve. Two common motions of playing tennis that can stress a tennis player's body are the swing of the racket and the side-to-side movement of the legs.

TENNIS ELBOW

Tennis elbow, or lateral epicondylitis, is pain and inflammation that occurs on the outside of the elbow. The most common cause of tennis elbow is overuse. Tendons at the end of the forearm muscles that attach to the lateral epicondyle become injured because of the repetitive stress of hitting thousands of tennis balls. Other contributing factors include age, not being accustomed to strenuous activity, decreased reaction time, and repetitive eccentric or elongating muscle contractions.

Treatment

The athlete lies faceup on the massage table with a bolster under the knees. The arms are at the side with the palms facing down. Lubricant is applied to the forearm from the wrist to the elbow using compressive effleurage 10 times. Next, compression strokes are applied from the elbow to the wrist three times. The trainer then applies Prossage Heat and stripping strokes from the wrist to the outside of the elbow three times. If the trainer locates any tender spots, she or he should apply direct pressure and hold for two to four seconds. Next, cross-fiber friction is gently applied to the outside of the elbow for 30 seconds. After a rest period of 1 minute, cross-fiber friction is again applied for 30 seconds. The trainer finishes the massage treatment by applying compressive effleurage 10 times.

To finish the elbow treatment, the athlete moves the wrist in flexion and extension, holding each position for two seconds and performing the action eight times. The athlete moves the wrist to the palm-up position and then the palm-down position, holding in each position for two seconds and performing the stretches eight times. If residual soreness is still present at the outside of the elbow, an ice pack can be applied for 20 minutes. A topical analgesic is then applied to the medial elbow. The analgesic can be applied three times a day every other day until the condition improves.

GROIN PULL

Groin pull, or adductor strain, is an injury to the inner thigh muscles. This injury occurs when the muscles of the inner thigh are overstretched. The adductor muscles are fan-shaped muscles located on the inner thigh that bring the legs together when they contract. Sudden movement in a side-to-side direction can strain the inner thigh, especially when the leg muscles are fatigued.

Treatment

The treatment starts with the athlete in the side-lying position and the bottom leg extended straight. The trainer applies massage lubricant to the inner thigh muscles from the knee to the hip with compressive effleurage 10 times and then applies petrissage to the muscles three times. Next, compression strokes are applied from the hip to the knee on the inner thigh three times. The trainer then applies Prossage Heat to the inner thigh and performs stripping strokes from the knee to the hip, applying direct pressure and holding for two to four seconds if any tender spots are located. To locate the exact site of a groin pull, the trainer has the athlete contract the adductors against resistance. Cross-fiber friction is applied to the exact site of the groin pull three times for 30 seconds, allowing a 1-minute rest after each application. The trainer adjusts the pressure of the cross-fiber friction to the athlete's comfort level. The massage ends with compressive effleurage strokes from the knee to the hip 10 times.

To finish the groin pull treatment, the adductors should be stretched. The athlete lies faceup, and the trainer brings the leg away from the midline of the body, gently stretches for two seconds, and returns the leg to the table. The adductor stretch should be performed eight times. If residual soreness is still present in the adductors, an ice pack can be applied for 20 minutes. Topical analgesic is then applied to the adductors. The analgesic is applied three times a day every other day until the condition improves.

Index

Note: The italicized *f* and *t* following page numbers refer to figures and tables, respectively.

A
Achilles tendon stretch 89
actin filaments 61-62, 62*f*
active isolated stretching 4, 72-74
active range of motion 13
adductor groin stretch 85
adductor strain 175
adjustable tables 19-20
agonist 43
anatomical planes 32*f*
anatomical range of motion 69
anatomical terminology 31, 31*t*-32*t*, 32*f*
anatomy
    joint 33-35, 34*f*-35*f*
    skeletal muscle 36-39, 36*f*-37*f*, 39*f*
ankle and calf stretches 88-90
antagonist 43
anterior lower-body postevent routine 112-113
anterior lower-body preevent routine 100-101
anterior lower-body recovery routine 138-142
anterior thighs, as common problem area 152-153
anterior upper-body postevent routine 105-107
anterior upper-body preevent routine 96-97
anterior upper-body recovery routine 127-132
arm extension stretch 78
arthritis 33
athlete
    interview of 5
    role of 9-10
atrophy 37-38

B
back
    as common problem area 154-155
    pain 172-173
    stretches 82-84
bag cover, for massage table 25-26
ballistic stretching 69
baseball, sport-specific treatments for 166-167
basketball, sport-specific treatments for 168-169
bathroom facilities 19
bent-knee hamstring stretch 85
bent-knee trunk flexion stretch 83
Biofreeze 23
body chart 5, 24, 52, 58, 120-121
bolsters 21, 29
bones 33
breathing 71
broadening strokes 14, 63-64, 103, 125
bunions 158-159
bursae 35, 35*f*

C
calf and ankle stretches 88-90
cartilage 33, 34*f*, 35
cervical extension 74
cervical flexion 74
cervical flexion with 45-degree head turn 75
cervical hyperextension with 45-degree head turn 76
cervical rotation 75
cervical stinger 164-165
chest stretch with arms extended 77
chest stretch with arms extended 45 degrees above shoulders 77
chest stretch with arms extended 45 degrees below shoulders 77
chondromalacia patella 160-161
circular friction 12, 92
circumduction of ankle 88
cleaning supplies 24, 28
cold therapy 22
common problem areas 149-156
compression strokes 13-14, 63, 92, 103, 123-124
compressive effleurage 13, 63-64, 102-104, 123
concentric contraction 38, 39*f*
continuing education 4-5
contraction types 38-39, 39*f*
contracts, for preevent massage 49-51
contusions 60
cool-down 59
cramps 40-41
creams 22-23
cross-fiber friction 14, 42, 122, 124
crush-proof containers 27-28
cycling, sport-specific treatments for 160-161

D
decorations 19
deep calf stretch for soleus 89
deep transverse friction. *See* cross-fiber friction
delayed onset muscle soreness (DOMS) 39-40
directional terminology 32*t*
direct pressure 14, 122, 124
direct pressure test 121-122
DOMS. *See* delayed onset muscle soreness
double-leg knee to chest 83
draping materials 21

E
eccentric contraction 38, 39*f*
elbow and wrist stretches 80-82
emergencies 51, 58
encouragement 54-55
enthesitis 45
enthesopathy 45
equipment and supplies
    bolsters 21, 29
    cleaning supplies 24, 28
    crush-proof containers 27-28
    draping materials 21
    for event massage 24-30, 26*f*
    first aid kit 23, 28
    for heat and cold therapy 22
    intake forms 24, 27, 52, 56, 58, 120
    massage tables 17-21, 25-26, 29
    in massage treatment room 17-24, 20*f*
    music 23, 29
    oils, lotions, creams, and ointments 22-23

equipment and supplies *(continued)*
  pillows 21
  protective coverings 27
  resistance bands 21-22
  rolling stool 21
  ropes 21-22
  sound system 23, 29
  supply cabinet and hamper 24
  tent 27
  trainer's personal supplies
    28-29
  weights 21-22
event massage. *See also* postevent
    massage; preevent massage
  checklist for 26*f*
  equipment and supplies for
    24-30, 26*f*
  planning and setup for 29
event meeting 30
eversion ankle stretch 90
external hip rotation stretch 87

F
fascia 36-37
fast-twitch Type II fibers 37, 37*f*
feet, as common problem area
    150-151
fight or flight syndrome 8
figure-four iliotibial band stretch
    86
first aid kit 23, 28
first-degree strains 40
flexibility 67-68
flooring 18
football, sport-specific treatments
    for 164-165
forearms, as common problem
    area 156
friction 13, 92
full-body chart 5, 52, 58, 120-121

G
gluteus maximus stretch 84
golf, sport-specific treatments for
    172-173
golfer's elbow 80, 156, 173
groin pull 175

H
hamper 24
hamstring strains 170-171
headrest 20
heat therapy 22
hip and knee stretches 84-88
hip flexor psoas stretch 86
hips, as common problem area
    153-154
hyaline cartilage 33, 35
hypertrophy 37-38

hypoxic injury 42

I
ice, application of 42
iliotibial band syndrome 161
inflammation 60
injuries
  discovery of, in preevent
    massage 56
  hypoxic 42
  management of 11-12
  recognition of, in postevent
    massage 60-61
  scar tissue and 41-42
intake information 5, 6*f*-7*f*, 9,
    24, 27, 52, 56, 58, 120
intent 11-12, 16, 49, 57, 70, 91,
    102
inter-competition massage 11
internal hip rotation stretch 87
interviews
  of athlete 5
  postevent massage 59, 64
  preevent massage 53-54
inversion ankle stretch 90
isometric contraction 38

J
jogger's heel 158
joints
  capsules of 34-35
  movement of 42-47, 44*t*, 46*t*
  ranges of motion of 45-47, 46*t*
  structural anatomy of 33-35,
    34*f*-35*f*
jostling 14, 92, 125
jumper's knee 168

K
knee and hip stretches 84-88
knee external rotation stretch 88
knee internal rotation stretch 87

L
lacerations 60
lateral flexion 75
lateral rotator shoulder stretch 78
lateral trunk side-bending stretch
    84
licensure 4-5
ligaments 35
lighting system 18
Ling, Pehr Henrik 3
logistical preparations
  for postevent massage 58-59
  for preevent massage 51-52
lotions 22-23
lower-body massage
  postevent 104, 112-117

preevent 55-56, 93, 98-101
  recovery 126, 138-147
lower legs, as common problem
    area 151-152
lubricants 22-23

M
maintenance massage 12
manufacturers' warranties 20-21
massage 3-4. *See also* sport
    massage
massage tables 17-21, 25-26, 29
massage treatment room
  checklist for 20*f*
  design of 17-19
  equipment in 17-24, 20*f*
Mattes, Aaron L. 4
Meagher, Jack 3-4
medial elbow tendinitis 166-167
medial rotator shoulder stretch 78
medical emergencies 51, 58
microtrauma 61-62
muscles
  anatomical terminology for 31,
    31*t*-32*t*, 32*f*
  contraction types and 38-39,
    39*f*
  in joint anatomy 33
  joint movement and 42-47, 44*t*,
    46*t*
  layering of 48
  pairings of 43-45, 44*t*
  problems with 39-42
  quality touch and 47-48
  skeletal 36-39, 36*f*-37*f*, 39*f*
  tissue texture and 47-48
muscle tendon units 33
music 23, 29
myosin filaments 61-62, 62*f*

N
neck strain 171
neck stretches 74-76
nonverbal communication 10

O
Oakworks massage tables 21, 25
oils 22-23
ointments 22-23
Olympic Games 3-4
on-site inspection 51
opposite arm flexion and
    extension stretch 76
overstretching 74

P
pain scale 8
pain spasm pain cycle 41
passive range of motion 13

percussion. *See* tapotement
personal space comfort zones 10
personal supplies, trainer's 28-29
petrissage 14, 63, 103, 123
pillows 21
planning
   event massage 29
   postevent massage 57-64
   preevent massage 49-56
portable tables 25-26
positions 9, 31*t*, 59
posterior hand touch 80
posterior lower-body postevent
     routine 114-117
posterior lower-body preevent
     routine 98-99
posterior lower-body recovery
     routine 143-147
posterior shoulder stretch 79
posterior upper-body postevent
     routine 108-111
posterior upper-body preevent
     routine 94-95
posterior upper-body recovery
     routine 133-137
postevent massage
   administering 104
   after massage 118
   cool-down and 59
   defined 12
   focus of 61-64
   injury recognition in 60-61
   intent of 11, 16, 57, 70, 102
   interview 59, 64
   logistical preparations for 58-59
   lower-body 104, 112-117
   planning 57-64
   precautions 57-58
   record-keeping preparations for
     58-59
   stretching in 64
   techniques 102-104
   upper-body 105-111
posttreatment suggestions 9-10
precautions, postevent 57-58
preevent massage
   administering 93
   after massage 102
   contracting for 49-51
   defined 11
   focus of 54-56
   injuries discovered in 56
   intent of 11, 16, 49, 70, 91
   interview 53-54
   logistical preparations for 51-52
   lower-body 55-56, 93, 98-101
   planning 49-56
   range of motion and stretching
     in 54

record-keeping preparations for
   51-52
   techniques 91-93
   timing for 52-53
   upper-body 55-56, 93-97
problem areas, common 149-156
Prossage Heat 22-23
protective coverings 27

Q
quality touch 47-48

R
range of motion
   active 13
   anatomical 69
   defined 68
   of joints 45-47, 46*t*
   passive 13
   in preevent massage 54
   techniques 14-15, 93, 125
reaction time 52
reciprocal inhibition 70
record keeping
   for postevent massage 58-59
   for preevent massage 51-52
   for recovery massage 120-121
recovery massage
   administering 126
   after massage 148
   assessment 120-122
   intent of 12
   lower-body 126, 138-147
   record keeping for 120-121
   techniques 122-126
   upper-body 126-137
referred pain 45
resistance bands 21-22
RICE 28, 61, 122
rolling stool 21
ropes 21-22
rotator cuff soreness 166-167
routines
   anterior lower-body postevent
     112-113
   anterior lower-body preevent
     100-101
   anterior lower-body recovery
     138-142
   anterior upper-body postevent
     105-107
   anterior upper-body preevent
     96-97
   anterior upper-body recovery
     127-132
   posterior lower-body postevent
     114-117
   posterior lower-body preevent
     98-99

posterior lower-body recovery
   143-147
posterior upper-body postevent
   108-111
posterior upper-body preevent
   94-95
posterior upper-body recovery
   133-137
runner's high 61
running, sport-specific treatments
    for 158-159

S
scar tissue 41-42
second-degree strains 40
shaking 13, 92, 125
sheets 21
shoulders, as common problem
    area 155-156
shoulder stretches 76-80
side-lying quadriceps stretch 86
side shoulder stretch 79
single-leg knee to chest 82
skeletal muscles, anatomy of
    36-39, 36*f*-37*f*, 39*f*
slow-twitch Type I fibers 37, 37*f*
soccer, sport-specific treatments
    for 170-171
sound system 23, 29
spasms 40-41
splinting 71
sport massage. *See also* event
     massage; postevent
     massage; preevent
     massage; recovery
     massage; routines
   checking results of 15
   defined 4-5, 51
   history of 3-4
   intent of 11-12, 16, 49, 57, 70,
     91, 102
   inter-competition 11
   introduction to 3-16
   key principles of 10-16
   maintenance 12
   as nonverbal communication 10
   process for 5-8, 6*f*-7*f*
   timing of 11-12, 16, 52-53
sport-specific treatments
   for baseball 166-167
   for basketball 168-169
   common problem areas for
     149-156
   for cycling 160-161
   for football 164-165
   for golf 172-173
   overview of 149, 157
   for running 158-159
   for soccer 170-171

sport-specific treatments *(continued)*
 for swimming 162-163
 for tennis 174-175
sprained ankle 169
sprains 61, 169
stabilizer 43
state regulations 4
static stretching 69
stationary tables 19-20
straight leg hamstring stretch 85
straight leg raise 73
strains 9, 40, 61, 170-171, 175
stretching
 active isolated 4, 72-74
 ankle and calf 88-90
 back 82-84
 ballistic 69
 benefits of 70-71
 breathing and 71
 consistent practice of 72
 fundamentals 68-70
 hip and knee 84-88
 neck 74-76
 overview of 67-68
 in postevent massage 64
 in preevent massage 54
 reciprocal inhibition 70
 shoulder 76-80
 static 69
 tense relax 69-70
 therapeutic 15, 93, 104, 125
 after treatment 9-10
 wrist and elbow 80-82
stripping strokes 14, 122, 124
subdeltoid bursa 35, 35f
superficial calf stretch for
 gastrocnemius 89
superstitions 53
supplies. *See* equipment and
 supplies
supply cabinet 24
Swedish massage 3
swimmer's knee 163
swimmer's shoulder 162-163
swimming, sport-specific
treatments for 162-163
synergist 43

T
tables, massage 17-21, 25-26, 29
tapotement 12, 92
tapping. *See* tapotement
 techniques
 broadening strokes 14, 63-64,
 103, 125
 circular friction 12, 92
 compression strokes 13, 63, 92,
 103, 123-124
 compressive effleurage 13-14,
 63-64, 102-104, 123

cross-fiber friction 14-15, 42,
 122, 124
direct pressure 14, 122, 124
friction 13, 92
jostling 13, 92, 125
overview of 12-15
petrissage 14, 63, 103, 123
postevent massage 102-104
preevent massage 91-93
range of motion 13, 93, 125
recovery massage 122-126
shaking 13, 92, 125
stripping strokes 14, 122, 124
tapotement 15, 92
therapeutic stretching 15, 93,
 104, 125
temperature 18-19
tender spots 9-10
tendons 33, 34f
tennis, sport-specific treatments
 for 174-175
tennis elbow 80, 156, 174
tense relax stretching 69-70
tent 27
therapeutic stretching 13, 93,
 104, 125
third-degree strains 40
timing 11-12, 16, 52-53
tissue texture 47-48
topical analgesics 23
touch comfort zones 10
trainer
 at event meeting 30
 honest relationship with 9
 personal supplies of 28-29
 quality touch and 47-48
 role of 8
treatments. *See* sport-specific
 treatments
triceps shoulder stretch 79
trigger points 9-10, 45, 67, 155
turf toe 164
Type I fibers. *See* slow-twitch
 Type I fibers
Type II fibers. *See* fast-twitch
 Type II fibers

U
upper-body massage
 postevent 105-111
 preevent 55-56, 93-97
 recovery 126-137
upper trapezius 155
upper trunk rotation stretch 83

W
warm-up 53
weights 21-22
Wellspring massage table 25

Western massage, earliest
 forms of 3
wrist abductor stretch 81
wrist adductor stretch 81
wrist and elbow stretches 80-82
wrist extensor stretch 81
wrist flexor stretch 80
wrist pronator stretch 82
wrist supinator stretch 82

About the Author

American Massage Therapy-certified sport massage therapist Michael McGillicuddy is a highly sought-after professional in his field. He has worked with numerous elite athletes and at national competitions for the Association of Tennis Professionals (ATP), the U.S. Figure Skating Association, U.S. Fencing, and at the Atlanta Olympic Games.

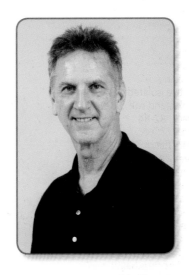

McGillicuddy graduated from the Florida School of Massage Therapy and is an approved provider for the Florida State Board of Massage Therapy and the national certification for massage and bodywork. His education has been shaped by leading sport massage therapists, including Benny Vaughn, Jack Meagher, Aaron Mattes, and Rich Phaigh.

McGillicuddy owns the Central Florida School of Massage Therapy in Winter Park, Florida, where he teaches and practices sport massage. He lives in Orlando, Florida.

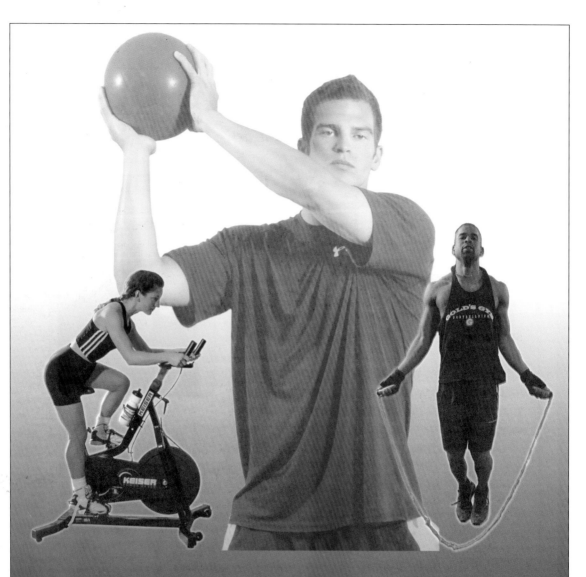

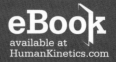